"Brian Jeansonne and I ̲   ̲   ̲   ̲ ̲ ̲ ̲ ̲ ̲ ̲
ALS, and because of our friendship and the wisdom and beauty in this book, I'm the luckiest man on the face of the earth. I just finished his book and I'm doing backflips on the inside. It's a post-graduate course on how to live in love with this crazy, wonderful Life. I'll read it again and again. Brian is my pastor, sojourner, and friend. I love him forever."

—**Steve Gleason, former New Orleans Saints player and founder of Team Gleason**

"With his mind firing, but his body failing, Brian Jeansonne contemplates his stories, where he came from, and where he wants to go in the time he has left. Alarmingly honest and hilariously down to earth, Brian Jeansonne's memoir asks the question: How do you move forward with a life full of circumstances and pitfalls you can't possibly control? Brian survives and even thrives by focusing full-throttle on the ever-narrowing avenues of possibility. While Brian's earthly body is permanently dormant, his entire life force is funneled into the furnace of his brain, where he is vibrantly alive. Cheeky, bawdy, courageous, contemplative, and full of tenderness for his family, neighbors, and humanity, Brian shines his light so we can see that on the open road and in the darkest corners, Love is Everywhere."

—**Jenifer Hixson, senior director,** *The Moth*

"Brian Jeansonne's book is an extraordinary achievement in itself, just the physical fact of it, in light of Brian's physical condition in year four of ALS. But the content is even more extraordinary. In one sense, the book reaches a summit of human transcendence over physical suffering, but in another sense, it does not strive for transcendence, instead dwelling wholly realistically on the brutalities and costs of this pernicious disease. At one level, the book is a bracing post-evangelical-pastor memoir; at another level, it is an ALS-journey memoir; at yet a third level, it is like reading the missing chapters of the Book of Job. The language of the book is extremely harsh, but the realities that language is trying to process are much harsher. I learned so much. Everyone should read this book."

—**Dr. David P. Gushee, distinguished professor of Christian Ethics, Mercer University**

"This book is insightful and poignant while being completely accessible and sometimes even raw. I cannot imagine all of the complexities of living with this diagnosis and accepting fate with open arms, but Brian can teach us all a thing or two about being authentic and accepting life and love with open arms. When it all comes down to it, love is the only thing that matters. Brian is right on. This book is for everyone!"

—**Julie Stokes, former Louisiana state legislator, nonprofit leader and entrepreneur**

"In *Onward Forward*, Brian gives us a masterclass on a life well-lived and well-loved. His close-up view of living with ALS is shared alongside the lessons he's learned in his roles as husband, father, pastor, coach, and teacher. Brian is able to strip away the rhetoric, the doctrine, and the bs to uncover the true purpose of life, which in its most raw form, is to love. There is a lesson for all of us in these pages."

—**Jennifer Fenton Weishaupt, founder, Ruby Slipper Cafe; adjunct professor, Freeman School of Business, Tulane University**

"Brian's raw story of the heartbreak, struggle, and loss of living with ALS is also a revelation of the deepened love, unexpected joy, and gratitude his diagnosis made possible. The view of life from Brian's power chair is a gift from this lovely, funny, often surprising book."

—**Dr. Stephen Kantrow, MD, pulmonary ALS specialist, professor of medicine, Louisiana State University**

BRIAN JEANSONNE
ONWARD FORWARD
MY JOURNEY WITH ALS

FINDING BEAUTY AND LOVE IN THE CLUSTERF*CK

FOREWORD BY: ALANIS MORISSETTE

Onward Forward-My Journey with ALS: Finding Beauty and Love in the Clusterfuck

Copyright © 2023 by Brian Jeansonne

All rights reserved. No part of this publication may be reproduced, distributed, or transmitted in any form or by any means, including photocopying, recording or other electronic or mechanical methods, without the prior written permission of the author, except in the case of brief quotations embodied in reviews and certain other non-commercial uses permitted by copyright law.

Without in any way limiting the author's [and publisher's] exclusive rights under copyright, any use of this publication to "train" generative artificial intelligence (AI) technologies to generate text is expressly prohibited. The author reserves all rights to license uses of this work for generative AI training and development of machine learning language models.

Printed in the United States of America
Hardcover ISBN: 978-1-961624-88-7
Paperback ISBN: 978-1-961624-89-4
Ebook ISBN: 978-1-961624-90-0
Library of Congress Control Number: 2024914280

DartFrog Blue is the traditional publishing imprint of
DartFrog Books, LLC.

301 S. McDowell St.
Suite 125-1625
Charlotte, NC 28204
www.DartFrogBooks.com

Dedicated to The Jeansonne 7
My wife, my best friend, and my person, Kristy
And to my children,
Micah, Jonah, Nate, Lucas, and Zoe Moon

"Now look, this is a sad moment right here, for all of us. There ain't nothing I can say standing in front of you right now that can take that away, but please do me this favor, will you? Lift your heads up, look around this locker room. You know, look at everybody else in here. And I want you to be grateful that you're going through this sad moment with all these other folks because I promise you there is something worse out there than being sad. And that is being alone and being sad. Ain't nobody in this room alone. Let's be sad now, let's be sad together, and then we [get back up]. Onward. Forward."
—Ted Lasso

TABLE OF CONTENTS

Foreword by Alanis Morissette 1
Introduction: The Beauty of Uncertainty 7
Chapter 1: ALS I 11
Chapter 2: On Journey 33
Chapter 3: On Oneness 55
Chapter 4: On Soul 65
Chapter 5: ALS II 75
Chapter 6: On Comparison 91
Chapter 7: On Suffering 101
Chapter 8: On Training 111
Chapter 9: On Presence 123
Chapter 10: ALS III 133
Chapter 11: On Contentment 155
Chapter 12: On Relationships 163
Chapter 13: On Conflict 177
Chapter 14: On Kids 191
Chapter 15: On Life 209
Chapter 16: ALS IV 223
Chapter 17: On Love 237
Appendix 01: A Letter to Those I Pastored 251
Appendix 02: The Gospel According to Ted Lasso* 255
Appendix 03: ALS Outtakes 257
Acknowledgments 267
About the Author 273

FOREWORD

BY ALANIS MORISSETTE

I first met Brian when an organization reached out to me to see if I would be open to connecting with him. When we met—initially over Zoom—I had no idea what to expect. Not knowing the degree to which we would be able communicate, I felt excited to just show up for him. I immediately saw that this would be unlike any experience I had had before. There was something in the quality of his groundedness. The way he held eye contact with me. With the silences between words allowing for a full-soul, no-turning-away kind of contact. An experience of pure presence. And while I may extoll the virtues of this quality of meeting, I was still scared of it. As brave as I might seem at times, I am still terrified of intimacy. It was like a "clear seeing" was happening when across from Brian, and had I not been doing inner work to build my fortitude with silence and all it asks of us, I might have shied away. With his wife, Kristy, by his side as the powerful superheroine that I have now come to know her as, I knew this wasn't a simple meeting of humans, but rather a meeting of two souls with a similar mission, albeit coming at it from unique angles.

Right out of the gate, Brian shared with me that he was attempting to chase and find the ultimate word to describe life and God and light. We laughed about how we both kept chasing the perfect word—the right languaging—to describe that felt sense of connection to *all*. I'd played with different wordings: light. The one permanent. Of course, God. Ultimately, I landed on the word that would become a starting point for me and Brian.

"I didn't know what to call it for a minute," he told me. "And then I saw that you used the word *Oneness* in your song "Ablaze"— '*keep your core connected to the Oneness.*'"

He said it just felt like the most appropriate word to use to describe something indescribable.

Ah, I had just met a brother. A lover of music, people, philosophy, life, and God—in all its "everythingness." A fully lit and very exciting soul. And a soul who clearly is living his vocation, having allowed his leadership role in life to expand as his life circumstances did.

Brian's formidable and intricate qualities of leadership became apparent the more we communicated. I quickly came to see that to know Brian is to be changed by Brian. Starting in his twenties, he had been a congregational leader, beginning as an evangelical pastor and evolving into a new understanding of spirituality and what matters most. Community, neighbors, friends, and family are at the center of Brian's life. He is a devoted father of five children and passionate husband to Kristy, all of whom you will come to know before you reach the last page of this book.

Although Brian's ALS diagnosis surely quickened his unfoldment as a leader, teacher, and guide, I also think there was an inevitability to his soul's evolution, and his own consciousness, that would have him arrive at this place no matter what his life circumstances were. From moment one, I was struck by the purity of being near him. Interacting with Brian, communicating with him, is like having a direct experience of a wise kindness. Spending time with him brings home the understanding that regardless of our physical limitations, and regardless of our physical capacities or aesthetic or talents, there is this deep, burning, warm soulfulness that permeates all of it—and Brian lives from that soul place.

That's not to say that he's not subject to his own humanity, because he is still a human being, and he shares this fact with a rawness and realness that is so intimate you can't help but embrace your own humanness much more readily alongside him. As you'll

FOREWORD

discover, Brian's fortitude and vulnerability are some of the many facets of his power.

Brian is a poet, a man of linguistic prowess and interpersonal and spiritual high intelligence. He is, archetypally, someone whom I want to follow into a towering inferno—because being on the receiving end of his attention will alchemically support you to be the person you were always meant to be.

At its bare essence, this is a book about allowing life to gently (and sometimes not so gently) catapult us into doing our soul work. Brian is the guide you will find yourself grateful to have by your side. As he will tell you himself, the journey of the soul is dangerous, thrilling, invigorating, fascinating, scary—and worth it.

* * * * *

Brian takes us on a journey—into his early days as a fervent young pastor and building a beautiful life with his love, Kristy, and their kids; and through the crucible of awakening that disease has rendered—where his unflinching honesty brings us right here, into this sacred moment. Challenge and tears and frustration and surrender and all.

Brian's searing and endearing sense of humor will lift you while he describes parts of his journey in his unique, conversational style. His love of life permeates the details. His positivity underpins his challenges and vulnerabilities in a way that has me hanging on to each word he shares. As he reflects back on key moments of his life, an astonishing thing happens. We get to experience the "past" with the same immediacy and aliveness as the present. Maybe this is because Brian holds it all with such full acceptance and gratitude. With a wholeness imperative that resonates with me on a profoundly deep level.

Early on, he tells us of the paradox he was living as he began to write: "Despite often being sad, I was grateful and excited about love and life. My life was a living, breathing juxtaposition."

Years before he was diagnosed with ALS, Brian had navigated through the dark waters of spiritual crises and depression. As he tells it, he had already "made it to the bottom" of his life, and so when a second opinion confirmed the diagnosis, he knew what to do: "I grabbed my pickaxe and my flashlight and got back to work…"

He asked himself the hard questions. No, the *hardest* questions. "How will I tell my kids? What will happen when I can't walk anymore? Or eat? Or speak? What will happen to Kristy and me? Who am I now? How will our family survive now that I can't work? What's my purpose? If I could be dead in two years, how should I spend my time? What's important?"

He was thrust into a deeper exploration of his interior life—examining every belief and choice along the way in. "Yes, I'm physically confined …," he says, "but emotionally and mentally I still have a choice." Brian's sense of freedom—beyond any perceived limitation—is one of the many inspiring parts of knowing him.

Throughout the pages of this book, Brian moves seamlessly between the roles of narrator of his own story and soul guide for those of us who are drawn here because we do not want to miss out on one more day of living with our hearts open wide. He knows that we, too, may be in the fire of our own loss or fear and therefore asks us to keep going, to persevere on behalf of love, no matter where we find ourselves today. He implores us to put one tender foot in front of the other, to pay attention, opening our eyes to the Oneness that we are an integral part of.

He takes us by the hand along the proverbial road less traveled—the path of complete and often messy surrender to love, letting go of attempting to control life so that we may actually experience it. He encourages us to go after this love at all costs, assuring us that we won't be disappointed. He reminds us that there is no greater gift in life than to be fully here for it. This beautiful man—who has lost and found and opened like a lotus flower to the wonder of it all—assures us of the things we have always wanted to be true, saying, "The world is full of life and love and magic for those who have eyes to see. Everything is alive with spirit and soul. We're integrally connected... There's no me without you. Everything is sacred and holy."

* * * * *

Today, whenever I interact with Brian, whether it's through a text or more directly, it is always an instant transmission of profound, knowing love. My day-to-day ego mind, and its many adorable and mundane considerations, takes a bow and steps quietly back in the face of that love. Something generous and wise is afoot. I always feel it when I connect with him. My wish is for you to feel it too, with me, here inside this blessed book.

Brian will remind you that our goal is not to create a life without problems, but instead to discover how to be fully engaged in our lives—in what he calls "the good, the bad, and the shitshow."

He will open your eyes to the truth that the world needs you. It needs your personal contribution, regardless of how large or small that may appear to be. And, yes, he will urge you to take care of your soul— including spending some time alone with yourself, sitting in the fertile silence. He will inspire you to *run* toward your "truest self" with total abandon, with your love blazing. And he will help you to feel a deeper sense of safety, assuring that your soul will not misguide you.

If you will pay attention to the signs Brian speaks of, to their music and invitations and musings, they will lead you to your life.

I picture Brian on his porch, in silence, BEING. And wherever I am on this planet, I picture myself sitting there next to him. Smiling. Basking in the warmth of presence, and quietly giggling to ourselves.

Meeting Brian and Kristy has been one of the greatest gifts of my life.

I am beside myself to introduce them to you too.
—Alanis Morissette

INTRODUCTION

THE BEAUTY OF UNCERTAINTY

"Be curious, not judgmental."
—Ted Lasso*

To make sense of my journey, you will need to know a few things about me. I was born in 1976 and raised right on the outskirts of New Orleans, Louisiana, in a little city called Kenner, which in many ways is like a foreign country compared to the city just twelve miles east. I lived there in the suburbs for my first thirty-eight years; since then, I've been lucky to live in the actual city of New Orleans—Bayou St. John, to be exact. One of the greatest places on earth.

I was raised in a Christian family, and my dad was a pastor. I chose the Christian path for myself when I was nineteen. After graduating from the University of New Orleans in 1999 at the age of twenty-two, I was hired as an associate pastor at my dad's church, where I served for seventeen years.

I married my wonderful Kristy in 2003 at the age of twenty-six, and together we created a beautiful family, four boys and one girl. Plus two dogs, whose names should be Yin and Yang. In 2016, when I was thirty-eight, Kristy, the kids, and I ventured out to start our own church in Midcity, New Orleans. We pastored that church for five years.

We were living our dream. Our family was thriving, and we were enjoying everything about life. Living in the city with five kids was expensive, so Kristy got a job as a producer's assistant, a job that afforded her the opportunity to still be with the family often. I was working four jobs, all of which still allowed me to be very present for my family, mostly because I made my own schedule.

Out of nowhere in 2020, we got sucker-punched when, at the age of forty-three, I was diagnosed with amyotrophic lateral sclerosis, or ALS, also known as Lou Gehrig's disease. ALS is a neurological disease that kills your motor neurons; in other words, the brain can still send commands to your muscles, but the muscles don't receive the information because the motor neurons are dead. Eventually ALS kills the muscles that enable you to swallow, and thus eat, and it kills the ones that enable you to breathe. This process takes anywhere from two to five years. Most doctors agree ALS is one of the cruelest diseases, as it's not only a death sentence—it destroys every part of your body before killing you. There is no treatment, only management.

My diagnosis was obviously a blow of magnificent proportions to our family. It would change everything for us. At the time we had no way of knowing that, in some ways, it would change our lives for the better. One thing you will notice in this book is that I don't use war language when I talk about ALS. I'm not fighting for my life or battling ALS or claiming victory. I'm a lover, not a fighter. Instead, I'm *journeying with* ALS.

One of my favorite books is *Letters to a Young Poet*, written by the poet Rainer Maria Rilke in the early 1900s. In this book, Rilke corresponds with a young aspiring poet by the name of Franz Xaver Kappus. In one letter, Rilke writes to Kappus,

> *Have patience with everything unresolved in your heart, and try to love the questions themselves, as if they were locked rooms or books written in a very foreign language. Don't search for the answers which could not be given to you, because then you would not be able to live them. And the point is to live everything. Live the questions now.*

THE BEAUTY OF UNCERTAINTY

I've always been inquisitive. I love questions. I love pushing the boundaries. At the age of three, probably my earliest memory, I was outside with my dad as he cut the grass. When he stopped for a water break, I made my way to the lawnmower and asked, "What is this?" Before he could answer, I reached for and touched the muffler and burned the skin right off my finger. In spite of this experience, I remained the kid who asked "why" about everything. I spent most of first, second, and third grades in the principal's office because I believed rules were made to be broken. As I got older, I continued my journey of inquisitiveness, questioning teachers and coaches and professors, as well as learning which rules could be bent, and which ones could be broken.

Living the questions has always been thrilling and life-giving to me. That includes during my twenty-two years of pastoring: I continued to ask questions. The struggle, as I would realize later, was that my questions didn't dig deep enough. Though I still loved investigating and remained curious, I held tightly to some deeply ingrained beliefs without question—political, religious, and moral beliefs. I have come to understand that changing our minds is one of the most difficult things for humans to do. It's also the only way we change and evolve and grow.

I'm convinced that of all the wrongs humans are capable of, the absolute worst wrong is certainty. A person who's certain of anything outside the laws of mathematics and science is dangerous. Hitler was certain. Alexander the Great was certain. George W. Bush was certain. Osama bin Laden was certain, as were the men who hijacked the planes on 9/11. Preachers and imams and rabbis and priests are certain. And we could go on and on.

I once heard the phrase, "be curious, not judgmental."*[1] It's often attributed to Walt Whitman, but I learned it from Ted Lasso.

---

[1] Throughout the book you will see asterisks; these gems are from Ted Lasso and his friends.

Whoever said it, I've taken it to heart. The problem with certainty, be it religious or ideological or political or moral, is that it robs us of our desire and need to be curious, and it destroys our ability to love. To truly love without condition. When we are certain, we are no longer curious, and we become judgmental. Again—I cannot say it enough—it's my opinion that certainty is the worst wrong. I'm almost certain of it.

I wrote a book in my mid-thirties. I read that book now and am so grateful I didn't publish it, as I no longer agree with 75 percent of it. Part of the reason I didn't publish it was that I noticed a pattern that my ideas about God, relationships, and more would change and evolve year to year; I decided I wouldn't write a book until I was at least fifty, maybe even sixty, when I imagined my thoughts and worldview would be more fixed. However, I'm now forty-seven, and I don't know that I will make it to fifty, and I definitely don't know that I will make it to sixty. It seems now's the time.

Through these pages, I will share some of my story, as well as my thoughts on suffering, love, life, contentment, comparison, God, and more during my dying years. In the event I do make it ten more years, expect a revised version of this book because I intend to keep learning and growing and evolving. What you hold in your hands is what I have concluded up to now. When it's all said and done, though, the truth is, I don't know shit about fuck.

Each of us is given this one life, this one opportunity to live and journey and experience the world in all its beauty. We each must make this journey. This is mine.

Life is a beautiful clusterfuck and love is here.
Onward. Forward.*
love.

CHAPTER 1

ALS I

"Welcome to earth,
Joy and strife,
Amazement and horror,
Will carve out your life."
—Anders Osborne; Welcome to Earth

I awoke at 6:30 a.m., as was my practice. It was September 2019, a typical warm morning in New Orleans. I dressed in my workout clothes and made my way to the family room. As I had every morning for the previous two years, I pulled out my workout mat and my dumbbells and hit play. Beachbody workouts afforded me the opportunity to work out at home. I rotated between p90x, p90x3, and Insanity; I was currently using the lift4 workout. (Pardon the lingo—fellow Beachbody enthusiasts will know.) I was in the best shape of my life. My hour-long workout was exhilarating. Afterward, I laced up my brand-new running shoes and headed out to christen them with a short three-mile run. The New Orleans Rock 'n' Roll Half Marathon was five months away, and I was beginning to train.

At the one-mile mark of my usual route along Bayou St. John, I noticed my gait was off: My left foot was not making its full stride through; it seemed to be dragging as it hit the dirt beneath my feet on its way forward. I thought very little of it, other than perhaps the new shoes weren't a good fit for me.

That afternoon, I walked about a mile and a half to my second job teaching PE to elementary school kids at Morris Jeff Community School. On this day, we played one of the kids' favorites, and mine too—dodgeball. As I walked across the gym to retrieve a ball, my left foot grabbed the gym floor, and I stumbled.

The next morning, after my usual early wake-up, I set to doing lunges with twenty-pound dumbbells. As I lunged forward with my left foot, I lost my balance and fell to the floor. Everything felt so awkward, and I wracked my brain trying to recall how I might have hurt myself. But that was just it: I was completely in tune with my body, and I knew I wasn't hurt.

Nevertheless, I laid off my foot so it could heal. As the weeks progressed, though, it didn't get better. As a matter of fact, I developed a slight limp. It wasn't really noticeable to others, but I could feel it. At this point I mentioned it to Kristy and asked if she could make me a doctor's appointment.

I believe—no, I know for a fact—that her reply was, "Boy, do I look like your secretary?"

I told her that was an outdated term. It's an administrative assistant.

I didn't even know where to start, so I called my dad who had a friend working at an orthopedic clinic. That November, I had an appointment. After I explained to the doctor what was going on, he had me walk the hall.

"You're right," he said. "You definitely have a limp, but I don't think this is orthopedic." He encouraged me to see a neurologist.

At this point I knew something was wrong, but I wasn't overly concerned. Maybe I'd had a minor stroke or agitated some nerves. The neurologist didn't seem too concerned either and told me to stop riding my bike, which was how I got everywhere, and come back in six weeks. During that time, my limp got worse. The doctor thought it wise to order some tests. So, I scheduled an MRI for my brain and back, as well as an EMG with my neurologist to evaluate the electrical activity produced by my skeletal muscles. The EMG showed minor nerve irritation, but the doctor wasn't concerned.

After about a week my MRI results showed no issues. My brain and spine were fine. I didn't know what else to do, so I quit worrying about it. My limp continued to worsen.

In February 2020, I went to the French Quarter with my son Nate, who was thirteen at the time, to see his fourteen-year-old brother, Jonah, march in a Mardi Gras parade with his school band. We had to park about fifteen blocks from the parade route. We clowned around with each other as we walked, and I noticed my limp getting worse. About six blocks from our destination, I tripped and sprained my ankle like I never had before. I writhed in pain on the ground as Nate did everything in his thirteen-year-old power to help until some passersby stopped and assisted me to a nearby stoop. I was on the verge of passing out from pain, but I knew I couldn't leave Nate to navigate the New Orleans streets by himself. Eventually I calmed down, and we hitched a ride back to our car.

After six months of letting me be my own admin, Kristy was frustrated and decided to take over. She scheduled an appointment for my ankle with an orthopedist who had done surgery on our oldest son's foot a few years earlier. He put me in a boot, and while there we asked him about my symptoms, which now included fasciculations in my right leg. He wanted me to see his associate who specialized in the back.

A week later, the back doctor looked at my MRIs and with great concern said, "This is not your back or brain." He gave us a name for a neuromuscular specialist.

When I asked him how concerned he was, he looked at me and said, "I'm not a neurologist, but I'm quite concerned. Maybe ALS concerned."

We were unable to get an appointment with the doctor he recommended, and then on Friday the 13th of March 2020, the world shut down due to the worldwide pandemic known as Covid-19. Doctor's offices. Grocery stores. Theaters. Restaurants. Churches. Jobs. Everything. Shut down.

By this time Kristy was concerned and started texting her people. Liz, who was a doctor in New York at the time. Ecoee, who was a well-known nurse in New Orleans. And others. Somehow the stars aligned; everyone had a connection to one neuromuscular specialist, Dr. Edwards. After reviewing all my medical records, doctor notes, and test results, Dr. Edwards asked to see us in person. That was April 14, 2020. Everything was still shut down. He had to turn the lights on at his office when we arrived. There was no administrative staff. No nurses. No other patients.

I wasn't nervous, as I had developed the practice of not worrying about things until they happened. After all, most of the things I ever worried about never came to fruition. I lived by the philosophy, "Find out before you flip out."* I sat on the exam table, and Kristy sat in a chair to my right. Dr. Edwards asked me a few questions about my symptoms and the history of my exploration into them.

He then examined my body for about four minutes, put down his instruments, and said, "Mr. Jeansonne, there's no easy way to say this. This is ALS. I'm so sorry."

Everything went silent. You know in movies when there's a loud explosion followed by a sharp, high-pitched sound, and the characters are talking but can't be heard? It was like that. Dr. Edwards was talking, but I couldn't hear anything, only saw his mouth moving. Tears were streaming down Kristy's face, but I had no idea why she was crying. I couldn't hear or feel. Everything was numb. After what seemed like half an hour—it was probably three minutes—Dr. Edwards suggested we get a second opinion, but he was 99.9 percent sure he was correct. He said we could have the room as long as we liked. We left immediately. As we entered the corridor, I fell to the ground, feeling like a piling in the shaft of a pile driver. I had been smashed to smithereens, and I wept in that corridor for what seemed like hours. Kristy had texted my parents, and by the time we composed ourselves and made it to the hospital lobby, my parents were there waiting for us. We told them the diagnosis, and the four of us sat quietly and wept there.

That afternoon, Kristy and I walked to the neighborhood park and sat together on an old, worn bench beneath a beautiful, great oak tree. We didn't talk; we held each other and cried and took ussies* to document the worst day of our lives. We knew Dr. Edwards was right but still scheduled our second opinion for a week later. During that week we sat with the news, only telling our closest people. We didn't tell our kids because, honestly, we didn't know how.

Just like Dr. Edwards, Dr. Rau turned the lights on for us. She examined my body for about twenty minutes and then looked me in the eye and said, "There's no easy way to say this, Brian. You have ALS. I'm so sorry."

As New Orleanians, we didn't need an explanation of ALS. Perhaps one of the most famous New Orleanians alive, Steve Gleason, has ALS. We understood the disease through his story and knew the grim prognosis. In 2016, I saw Steve's documentary, *Gleason*, in the theater. I remember sitting there after the credits rolled, just weeping.

The night of the documentary as we lay in bed, I said to Kris, "There are a lot of ways I don't want to die, but ALS is at the top of my list." I knocked on the headboard of our bed, but it was from IKEA and turned out to only be faux wood.

Oof.

The next morning as I sat on my porch with my coffee, I journaled,

August 30, 2016

There are a few movies that have greatly impacted my life, movies that tell stories that reset or reorient my internal compass. Yesterday, I saw one of those movies and I am still reeling from it, processing what it means for me.

The movie was Gleason—*the story of former New Orleans*

> Saints player Steve Gleason, who was diagnosed with ALS in 2011.
> Faced with his own mortality and a timeline for his own life, Gleason—through the wonderful highs and excruciating lows—strives endlessly to be present each moment, making the most of each day.
> I'm not sure all of the ways this story will shape me, but I do sense deeply that the words "Do not worry about tomorrow, for tomorrow will worry about itself" are for me right now.

As much as I was taken by Steve's approach to ALS, I was even more struck by his wife, Michel's, attitude, courage, honesty, and rawness. In referring to ALS near the end of the documentary, Michel utters the words, "It's a motherfucker." That phrase stuck with me and seemed the most appropriate term for such a disease.

We began telling people and prepared to tell our kids, who were eight, eleven, thirteen, fourteen, and fifteen years old at the time. That was perhaps the worst day of my life, maybe even worse than the day I was diagnosed. We asked the three older boys to join us on the porch, deciding Lucas and Zoe Moon were too young for this conversation. We spoke to them later, two on one. As we sat on the porch with the boys and began fumbling with our words, I lost all composure and began to sob, so much that Kris had to finish telling them.

We did not tell the boys about the terminality of the disease, but they knew about Steve Gleason, so they understood what was to come. It was interesting to watch how each child responded. Micah (15) became very angry and worked through his frustration by retreating to a fantasy world of comics and superheroes in which he created his own superhero and eventual comic book. Jonah (14) became busy, always on the go, not wanting to be home. Nathan (13) immediately began working out in preparation for the day he would need to pick me up. Lucas (11) and Zoe Moon (8) just continued with life. I think they were too young to comprehend the true nature of the situation.

Apparently, ALS is a big deal because my doctors had me meet with both physical and occupational therapists within two weeks of diagnosis. Both of them examined me and talked to me about what was going on with my body and what I might expect in the near future. Unbeknownst to me, they had arranged for a wheelchair rep to walk me through options. Keep in mind that Kris was in the car, waiting, because the world was broken and no one was allowed to accompany me during the appointment. So, here I am, sitting scared in this clinic, and this guy starts talking to me about wheelchairs. He was so nonchalant, acting like this was normal, everyday conversation. I was just diagnosed two weeks earlier, and this guy is acting like it's no big deal. I hated it, and I hated him.

I started bawling, and the asshole just kept talking until my PT stepped in to say, "That's probably enough for today." My whole world was imploding, and I didn't know what to do.

I left the physical therapy appointment with a cane, to help with balance. I had barely processed my diagnosis. How was this happening already? The cane did make walking a bit easier, and I admit I liked the vibe. I already smoked a pipe, wore a porkpie hat, and sipped bourbon, so the cane seemed to complete the look. I got online and ordered a cane that better fit my style.

Within days we had friends talking over plans for remodeling our home to make it handicap-accessible. They discussed installing a lift on the side of our house, widening doorframes for a wheelchair, and completely renovating our primary bathroom.

I didn't understand; I only had a limp. But everyone else seemed to think we should start making moves. All I could think was, *Fuuuck!* I'd been writing poetry for years, so that evening I sat on my porch with a cigar and my bourbon, and I took the opportunity to express my feelings by penning perhaps my greatest poem to date:

Fuckity fuck, fuck, fuck.
Fuckity fuck, fuck, fuck.
Fuckity fuck, fuckity fuck.
Fuckity fuck, fuck, fuck.
Fuck!

Kristy and I were still pastoring the small church we started in 2016. I loved the forty people and wanted to pastor them as long as I could with integrity. Due to Covid, we were already meeting online in a Zoom room, so it was easy for me to keep going. The only thing I liked about Christianity by this time was Jesus because he seemed to be the only genuine part of the faith. So, I told the church we would read through the book of Luke and talk about Jesus. Period. I couldn't do anything more.

Kristy and I felt lost, and at the same time we sensed a deep peace. We went to bed laughing together as many nights as we did crying. We were scared, angry, sad, and distraught, and yet falling more and more in love, pressed against the wall and consciously choosing one another in sickness.

In June, we were directed to attend our first ALS clinic at Ochsner Medical Center. We had no idea what to expect. Turns out there was nothing to be afraid of. The purpose of the clinic is to afford ALS patients an opportunity to visit quarterly with each member of their care team in a single appointment. In just one four-hour visit, in one place, we met with all of my doctors, as well as my physical therapist, occupational therapist, speech-language pathologist, social worker, and dietitian. This would become our safe place where we could breathe, ask questions, and feel supported. Our first time at the clinic we met Dr. Kantrow, my pulmonologist. This man was the kindest, most empathetic man I had ever met. That day he gave me his cell phone number and told me to call him anytime I had a question, or if I just wanted to have a cup of coffee. I didn't know it at the time, but Dr. Kantrow would be the doctor to walk this entire journey with me.

Things progressed quickly. One afternoon, I got a visit from my new friend, Blair. Blair works for Team Gleason, a nonprofit organization that Steve Gleason founded upon his diagnosis with ALS in 2011. Team Gleason does many things, but its primary focus is to provide technology that helps people with ALS thrive.

Blair showed up at my house with a small, battery-powered wheelchair called the Jazzy. The Jazzy enabled me to conserve energy, as I found myself getting fatigued very easily.

Concurrent with the rush of difficult adjustments, some wonderful things were happening. One night, I arranged for Kris and myself to eat at one of our favorite neighborhood restaurants, Santa Fe on Esplanade Avenue. After dinner, I took her to nearby City Park, where, as a favor to me, friends had set up a blanket laid out with rose petals and wine and cheese at one of our favorite spots under the magnificent oaks. We sat for hours talking about our life together, listening to music, and laughing and crying together. As our evening progressed, one of our favorite songs, "Perfect" by Ed Sheeran, came on, and I asked Kristy if she would dance with me in the twilight. It took me about two full minutes to get up off the blanket, but I grabbed my cane and we danced together and held one another as though it were the first time we had ever embraced. As the song concluded, I got down on one knee and pulled a ring out of my pocket. I asked Kristy if she would marry me all over again.

This was a special ring in more ways than one. Kristy had been ringless for more than ten years, as we'd sold her original engagement and wedding rings in our quest to adopt our daughter Zoe Moon from Ethiopia. In addition, this was an uncut, unpolished diamond. To most, this would not be a pretty ring, but for Kristy and me this ring represented everything we were together. Raw.

Unpolished. Ragged. Worn. Tried. And yet, forged, enduring, strong, and unshakable.

Two weeks later, Kristy surprised me with a vow renewal and party with fifty of our closest friends under the same great oaks in City Park—on the hottest day in the history of ever. Beneath those sacred trees, on that hallowed ground, we once again vowed our lives and love to one another. It felt different from seventeen years earlier; there was more life and substance behind our words this time.

As beads of sweat rolled down our faces and our eyes filled with tears, Kristy vowed:

> *Today and every day,*
> *You are my best friend,*
> *My person.*
> *My promise to you is simple ... you are my one and only. My partner and my best friend.*
> *I will see you and hear you, I will fight for you and I will be honest with you.*
> *I will trust you and respect you, and I will never give up on you.*
> *I promise ... to dream with you, to have fun with you, to laugh with you, to cry with you.*
> *I promise to be with you in the good times and the bad.*
> *When we have a lot, and when we have a little. When we are healthy and when we are unwell.*
> *No matter what happens to us in the future, every day we are together is the greatest day of my life.*

I hadn't been told to prepare, as that would have ruined the surprise, so I was left to recite traditional vows during the ceremony. I wrote these vows and recited them to her a few days later:

> *I choose you, this day and every day.*
> *I promise and desire to love you without end, without condition, without reciprocation.*
> *To honor you by listening to you, by supporting you, by asking what honors you.*
> *To make sure you know you are the most beautiful, lovely, merciful, kindhearted, badass woman alive.*
> *I promise to stay by your side when we have a lot and when we are just barely scraping by. In the really fun exciting times, and in the really mundane boring times. On the easy days and on the awful ones. When our health is good and thoughts of illness are unrealistic and ... when the wheels fall off and everything we felt for our future comes crashing down. I promise to learn to love you more beautifully each day, better than the one before.*
> *All of these things I desire to give to you for every single day of the rest of my life.*

Following the vow renewal, another 100 friends joined us for a party at our favorite brewery, Second Line, which Kristy had rented. We danced (I hobbled) and laughed and drank and sweated with our friends for hours. This was joy and love at its finest.

The next day Kristy and I left for California. Our goal was to make the trip as fun and lighthearted as possible. We knew the reality of our future, and we wanted to be fully present to one another and the moment. We landed in San Francisco, where we rented a white Mustang convertible with a trunk just big enough to fit my snazzy Jazzy wheelchair. *Actually* fitting the Jazzy into the trunk was a science, a bit like trying to fit OJ's hand into the glove. Again and again, as we spent fifteen days driving the Pacific Coast Highway down to San Diego, Kristy had to fold up the sixty-five-pound chair and squeeze it in there.

In San Francisco, we enjoyed Fisherman's Wharf, the seals, the clam chowder, and—the best part—the day we rented one of those three-wheeled go-carts and cruised the city streets. We also drove across the Golden Gate Bridge with the top down and continued north to see the redwoods. We felt like kids on our honeymoon, and it was magic.

After the Bay Area, we made our way south to Big Sur National Park for two nights. There was no Internet, and hiking wasn't an option, so we had two solid days of nothing but each other. We bought a nice bottle of bourbon and spent the days sitting on the porch and talking as we took in the breathtaking views; at night we got drunk and played incredible sex games. Sorry, that's all you get! We knew in the back of our heads that our sex life would soon change, so we thoroughly enjoyed ourselves.

Continuing south, in Santa Barbara we hit up a great weed dispensary and stayed at this cute hotel right on the ocean that had a beautiful courtyard where we got high and enjoyed the boardwalk, the water, the weather, and each other. It might be important to mention something about my weed use here, as weed plays a significant role in my ALS journey. Before ALS, I only occasionally smoked marijuana, enjoying it on personal retreats or occasionally with a friend. Upon my diagnosis, at the height of Covid, I decided to smoke as often as I could. At my first clinic visit, one of my doctors encouraged me to use it for anxiety. I said, "Say less"—a doctor's order was all the convincing I needed. The weed did have some medicinal value, in that it helped my body relax and aided sleep, but mostly I just liked getting high. That's how marijuana became part of my daily routine for the first three years of ALS.

After Santa Barbara we made a pit stop in Los Angeles, where we connected with a few friends, and then finally landed at Coronado Bay in San Diego. As we pulled up to our hotel in Coronado Bay, I had to pee so badly we didn't have time to wrangle with Jazzy, so I grabbed my cane and started to hobble to the bathroom. Unfortunately, the bathroom was about two miles from the check-in desk. Halfway there I told Kris I didn't think I could make it, so she hoisted me from under the shoulder and assisted me the rest of the way. As soon as I got to the door, I peed all over myself. This was the first of many accidents. I was so embarrassed, distraught, and sad as I broke down crying, falling to the floor right outside the men's bathroom. Kristy happened to have a blanket with her, so she wrapped me in it and held me, and we cried on the floor together. It was a sobering moment as we realized how my disease was affecting me. We had spent the past eleven days living alongside the disease, not dwelling on it, and in this one moment it snuck up from behind and knocked us on our butts. We cried, got me changed, and got back on the horse. We were determined not to let ALS have the final word on this trip.

We spent the last four days of the trip in Coronado Bay. When it was time to fly home, we decided we weren't done. Instead, we canceled our flight and took three days to drive home with the top down. It was the best vacation of our lives.

On our way home, we got a call that the kids had been exposed to Covid. Keep in mind this was June 2020. We still didn't know much about the virus, so when we arrived home, I immediately moved in with our neighbor Margo, while Kristy quarantined with the kids for two weeks. I hadn't been with the kids for eighteen days. Though I was just next door and could talk to them from a "social distance," I couldn't hug them or hold Kristy. Every night before bed they called me and we would look through the windows at each other. It was incredibly difficult for all of us, but after two weeks everyone was in the clear; I moved back home, and we had a huge celebration with a family dinner, movie night, ice cream, and lots of hugs.

As the months passed, I continued to lose function in my legs. I began falling, once in the bathroom with no one around. It took me twenty minutes to get myself up. I knew my walking and standing days were nearing an end. By October, six months post-diagnosis, I was in my power chair full-time in the house. My power chair is an incredible piece of machinery and can be yours for just $50K. Power chairs are designed for quadriplegics and other people who can't move. My power chair is like a La-Z-Boy on wheels, only not as comfortable, though they make the chair as comfortable as possible since you'll be living in it. It's able to recline; I can lie flat; I can elevate my feet. In addition, my chair has an elevator that will elevate me to about five feet, eight inches tall, so when in conversation with someone I can be at eye level. The seat has a gel pad that forms to my butt. The chair can go up to six miles per hour and turns on a dime. If I didn't have ALS and had an extra fifty grand to blow, I'd probably get one just for the perks, like great seats at the theater, or getting ushered to the front of the line at amusement parks.

I could still make slight maneuvers myself, such as moving from my chair to the sofa or getting myself on the toilet, but anything that required steps was a no-go. If we wanted to leave the house, I had to transfer to my Jazzy, which was incredibly inconvenient because we didn't yet have a handicapped accessible van. Going anywhere became a chore, as Kris and the kids had to put me in and take me out of the car.

I could no longer get in bed by myself either. Kris and the kids needed to transfer me from my chair to the bed. My core strength was weakening, so I could hardly help them. This progression was a sobering reality check. Adding to the stress, sleeping became difficult—for both of us. I had always been a side-sleeper, but I couldn't easily get on my side by my own strength, so I would wake Kristy throughout the night to adjust and roll me. Things were getting very difficult very quickly, and I was losing my independence.

In September my friend of more than twenty years, Emmily, offered to stretch me three times a week. Emmily is an occupational therapist, so she understands the body and what I needed. Every Monday, Wednesday, and Friday, she got me to the floor, put on meditation music, and stretched my body for an hour. She created a beautiful, sacred space for us to share. Besides my family, Emmily was the only person with a front row seat to my progression. She always showed up with tenderness and love.

In November 2020, a group of friends gifted all seven of us a trip to Disney World. Two friends came along to help. The trip was incredible, and there were perks to being in a power chair: We got to bypass many of the lines, and we often got to ride rides two times in a row. Whether at Space Mountain, the Rock 'n' Roller Coaster, or the Teacups, my friend Shawn picked me up out of my chair and put me on the ride. Many of the rides were uncomfortable, as my core muscles were weakening and I was tossed about like a ragdoll, but I enjoyed every second of it.

One day at Animal Kingdom, I was hanging out drinking my third sixteen-ounce beer and watching the monkeys while everyone else was off riding rides. I was feeling pretty good. Then, as had become a normal occurrence, I suddenly had to pee. I had agreed not to leave that spot without assistance, but I really had to go, so against orders I drove myself to the bathroom. En route, I realized I didn't just feel good—I was wasted! Driving a wheelchair with ALS through Animal Kingdom while wasted and trying desperately not to pee your pants is no easy task. Eventually I found the nearest bathroom and rolled right up to the urinal. I grabbed the hardware to the urinal and tried to pull myself up, but the beer was too fast, and … I peed my pants. Once again, I was embarrassed and sad, but I was also drunk, and when I'm drunk everything is funny.

My phone rang.

"Hello."

It was Kristy. "Where are you?"

"I'm in the bathroom. I peed my pants."

"Which bathroom?"

It's a big park. I was wasted. "The men's bathroom."

She didn't find it as funny as I did. Eventually two of my boys located me, and we were all reunited. Shawn bought me a new shirt, and I spent the rest of the day in pee-soaked pants. No one else in the family found it as funny as I did, because no one else was forty-eight ounces of beer in. And that was the last time we ever went anywhere without a backup set of clothes.

While at Disney World, we received a message that the husband of a dear friend in Dallas, Jennifer, had had a seizure, fallen in his driveway, and smashed his head. He was on life support. They didn't think he would survive. As soon as we got back to New Orleans, we repacked, switched chairs to the Jazzy because it was easier for travel, headed back to the airport, and boarded a plane for Dallas. We spent two nights with Jennifer, time we're so grateful to have had, and her husband died soon after.

On our way home, as we sat eating at the airport, I suddenly had to take a crap. I wheeled myself to the bathroom and maneuvered myself onto the toilet on time, but as I tried to transition back into my chair I got stuck in an awkward, painful position between the toilet and the stall wall. A custodian who was fortuitously in the bathroom heard me yelling for help and got Kristy, who unstuck me, put my pants back on, and got me back in my chair. Another moment of facing the harsh reality that I was losing function at a very quick rate.

By December, eight months post-diagnosis, our lives had changed incredibly. I could no longer drive. For our entire marriage we had tag-teamed. Kristy would take this one to baseball while I would take another one to gymnastics. I would pick another up from art school while she would get dinner ready for all seven of us. I would help this one with homework while she took another one to tutoring. With five kids it was full-time from sunup until after sundown for both of us. With me out of the equation, Kristy was drowning.

Well, I wasn't exactly out of the equation. More like it, I had become the equation's X factor. In many ways, I had become a sixth child. Kristy would wake early to get ready so she could then get me out of bed, help me on and off the toilet, help me shower, help me get dressed, and finally put me in my chair. I could see how exhausted she was, which hurt. I felt like Benjamin Button, physically regressing and becoming more and more like an infant. And we hadn't even hit the difficult part of the disease yet.

And at the same time, so much love lightened our load. Immediately upon my diagnosis, our community began providing dinner for us. They did this five nights a week for the first two years, and in year three they continued to provide dinner twice a week. Then, in December 2020, my mom and a friend of ours started a grassroots campaign to raise money for a $60,000, twelve-passenger Ford Transit passenger van outfitted with a wheelchair lift that would fit our family of seven. That same month, a van was delivered to our home paid in full. Never underestimate the beauty and generosity of humanity. As I have come to believe, the world is full of magic, and people are amazing. The van enabled me to leave the house and maintain some normalcy in life. The van also enabled us to continue taking family road trips.

By January, I had plateaued: The disease progression slowed, and I found reprieve for about three months.

Though the disease was wreaking havoc on my body, it wasn't wreaking havoc on my spirit. Outside had always been my sanctuary, so I continued to roll myself eight blocks to CC's, my favorite coffee shop, situated on a beautiful stretch of Esplanade Avenue. I sat there for hours under the magnificent oaks and enjoyed my coffee. I also spent time sitting beneath cypress trees beside a lagoon at City Park. And, of course, I sat on my own front porch. My porch wasn't available during afternoon hours, though, because the sun was a scorcher. Fortunately, our neighbor Margo has an amazing side porch protected from the sun that I absolutely love. For years I'd sat on her porch while she was at work and I worked from home. In February 2021, once I could no longer walk, Margo had a wheelchair ramp installed so I could continue hanging on her porch. People are pure magic and love is everywhere.

Yes, that first year of ALS was a whirlwind for us, physically, spiritually, emotionally, mentally, vocationally, and socially.

Physically

ALS is known for the physical toll it takes on a person; for the casual observer, that's all there is to it. In my first year I lost the use of both legs and most of my left hand. Between April and December, I lost my ability to walk. That blew me away. I thought I would have more time than that. The physical losses were earth-shattering: to no longer be able to throw the football with my kids or coach baseball or walk to my coffee house or take my kids out for birthday breakfast. It all happened so fast. From the cane to a zippy wheelchair to a power chair to complete immobilization, all within one year, was devastating. I never imagined the disease would rob me of the simple pleasure of walking my dog so quickly.

I remember one day in February 2021 feeling like my chair had become a prison. Kristy was ready to get me up one morning, and I said, "Fuck the chair! I'm staying in bed."

That was my way, my only way, of sticking it to the chair. The physical toll was relentless, and it was only just starting. ALS really is a motherfucker.

Spiritually

Many may think that my spirituality changed because of ALS, but the truth is my views on spirituality had been changing for more than a decade; ALS gave me the freedom and time to accelerate that process. I write about this more extensively later in the book, but suffice it to say spirituality played a huge part in that first year and has continued to hold a very intimate space in my journey. In truth, spirituality is what has kept me in the game of life.

Emotionally

How does someone even begin to express the emotional weight that accompanies such a diagnosis? I was a wreck for the first few months. I felt like my life was over, I didn't know which way was up, and worst of all, I felt like I was drowning. Each night I sat on my porch and smoked a bowl or two as I tried to relax and make sense of this new world I had wandered into. Some nights, many nights, I sobbed uncontrollably for hours. I've always been a crier, even crying at Hallmark commercials, but this was a cry from the deepest parts of my being. Eventually, I was able to move through this phase of uncontrollable wailing on the regular, but the pain still visits from time to time.

That first year, I also experienced incredible moments of peace and joy and happiness and life. Kristy did too. We couldn't explain it or wrap our heads around it, but we were in it together, and we made a decision early on that we wouldn't live in fear of the future but instead live present in the day we were given; whatever feelings that day brought, we would embrace.

Mentally

What a mindfuck. One day you're living like you're invincible, and the next day you're told to get your affairs in order because you'll probably be dead in the next two to five years. All my hopes and dreams for the future were destroyed. Like seeing my kids graduate from high school, or one day seeing the adults they'll become. Even harder, my dreams of growing old with Kristy—decimated. It was a year of untangling these webs in my mind. The truth is none of us is guaranteed tomorrow, but I had certainly lived as if I were. As the first year progressed, I did come to grips with my own mortality; this was one of ALS's gifts.

Vocationally

This arena was easier for me. For years I felt myself drifting further and further from pastoring a church. The year before my diagnosis, I had picked up three additional jobs to help support our family. I drove for Uber from 4–8 a.m. a few mornings a week, and then for a few hours after the kids went to bed on weekends. I also worked part-time as a PE teacher and had two of my kids in class. Finally, I started a business called Seeds and Souls for which I would sit with people and help them explore the questions of soul and their inner life.

These avenues created extra income for our family, though my ultimate desire was to find a way out of leading a church. Exactly thirteen months after diagnosis, we closed the doors of the church we had spent five years pastoring. The only difficult part for me was losing the congregation I loved dearly. But it was necessary physically, mentally, and spiritually. I sensed that where I was going spiritually, these people couldn't follow. I knew I was leaving the well-worn path of the church as I had known it, and I didn't want to cause them to question or sway them in their own journey.

Socially

It's difficult to know how ALS impacted us socially, as Covid had broken social structures just one month prior to my diagnosis. We already weren't hanging out with most of our friends and loved ones. We did have a small neighborhood pod, which proved to be exactly what our family needed. For four months we spent every day on Margo's porch with our other neighbors, Stephanie and Merry. We ate dinner together every night. Margo taught my thirteen-year-old how to cook while Stephanie taught my eight-year-old how to say, "Shut the fuck up, bitch." Well, she didn't intentionally teach her, but Zoe Moon is a sponge. So, when she one day told me to, "Shut the fuck up, bitch," I didn't ground her but instead walked across the street and asked my sixty-two-year-old-neighbor for her phone and grounded her. Margo's porch was our sanctuary in a time of great uncertainty and turmoil. As the year moved on and Covid lightened up, we began to have porch nights with other friends. These were moments we cherished in our hearts, as we knew hangouts were numbered.

In that first year, I sat on my porch alone almost every single night, often into the early morning hours, with my weed and my thoughts. My life was coming to an end, and I had questions. I asked questions about everything. Everything. Nothing was off-limits. Nothing. Nothing was sacred. And everything was sacred. My time and thoughts were devoted to thinking on things of the soul, God, and the journey of my life—what had led me to this place.

That first year was a motherfucker, and yet something unexpected sprang forth from the soil of our pain: The seven of us began to grow stronger and closer. We were all in and committed to each other. Everyone took part in the bedtime routine, and we spent countless nights enjoying one another's company in ways we'd never done before. It was beautiful to behold. We spent our time being sad together, and then we gathered ourselves and chose to move onward, forward together. For years our family hashtag had been #thejeansonne7. At the end of year one, #thejeansonne7 was a force of love to be reckoned with. It led me to truly believe that beauty could rise from the ashes.

Or, as I like to say ...

Life is a beautiful clusterfuck and love is here.
Onward. Forward.*
love.

CHAPTER 2

ON JOURNEY

> *"I think things come into our lives to help us get from one place to a better one."*
>
> —Ted Lasso*

I've met a number of people who have made the five-hundred-mile pilgrimage across Spain to walk the Camino de Santiago. Some have done it as part of their midlife crisis, others as a spiritual pilgrimage, and others to refind their center. Their tales of experiencing parts of themselves they didn't even know existed are inspiring. And just as Frodo came face-to-face with the darkest parts of himself on the way to Mordor, forever changed, so they came back different too. That's what journeys do to people. They change you. If you let them.

One woman's Camino story in particular left an indelible mark on my soul. Every pilgrim is invited to leave something behind after their journey. As she stood at the end of the five-hundred-mile route, she experienced the soil beneath her feet changing from hard dirt to soft sand to frigid ocean waters. At that moment she realized her faithful, trustworthy boots that had been with her for every step and had stuck with her through thick and thin—they couldn't help her on the next leg of her journey.

So, she left her boots behind.

I've never traveled the Camino de Santiago, but I've come face-to-face with my truest self, as well as my shadow self. I've also learned how to care for and listen to my soul, and I am who I am today because of it. On my soul journey, I wore Converse. This is the story of my pilgrimage.

Part I: Being Formed - Decade I

My mom was raised in a strong Baptist tradition. My dad was raised nothing. Somewhere along the way, they chose to travel the Baptist path together. Growing up, I was immersed in the Baptist tradition, attending Sunday school and church on Sunday mornings and Sunday nights, as well as Wednesday nights. As if that wasn't enough, I went to the Christian school attached to the church on weekdays. This was the context for the indoctrination pool I would swim in for my first nine years. It was here I learned some fundamental lessons, such as God is a safe and loving father; Jesus, God's only son, died on a cross and came back to life; and everyone who says they believe this story will go to heaven when they die, while nonbelievers will go to a hell of fire. Believing all of the above was critical, we were taught, because everyone is born with a sinful heart, we are evil by birth, and we must ask for forgiveness and be washed clean. I also grew up learning the Bible is a factual, perfect book. All the cool (to a young boy) and terrifying stories of the Old Testament were essentially saying you'd be fine if you were on the right side of God but, as the Irishman would say, you'd be fucked if you found yourself on the wrong side.

At age seven, I was baptized, which means I asked Jesus into my heart and now was forgiven for my sins and guaranteed a cloud in heaven. I've raised five kids, which means I've raised five seven-year-olds, none of whom was ever bad enough to spank, let alone bad enough to be banned to a fiery hell. So, why would a seven-year-old get baptized? Indoctrination.

My memories of my early Baptist upbringing can be summed up in one story. Have you ever heard the one about how God freed his people out of Egypt and then annihilated their enemies—the Egyptians—by luring them into an open sea and then causing the sea to close, thus drowning thousands and thousands of human beings? God's drowning his enemies made sense at the time, as we had already learned about how he once decided to drown the entire population of Earth, minus one guy and his family.

Anyway, we learned about the destruction of the Egyptians the day my second-grade teacher used a large pan of blue Jell-O to turn an entire classroom into God-fearing eight-year-olds—and by God-fearing, I mean literally fearful of God. She had carefully unmolded a rectangle of Jell-O on a piece of tinfoil cut right down the middle. Then, during Bible story time, as she read from the book of Exodus, she pulled the tinfoil in opposite directions, which literally divided the blue Jell-O Red Sea in half! At that point she allowed some of us to march little paper characters we'd made through the Jell-O waters onto dry land. We were the chosen ones freed from Egypt. Meanwhile, a group of our friends had created little paper chariots and soldiers, the Egyptian Army. When it was their turn to chase our cute little Israelite paper people across the Jell-O Sea, our teacher let go of the tinfoil, which caused the Jell-O in all of its blue fury to crush and drown the chariots and soldiers. It was so violent; you could almost hear the paper people screaming for their lives. This was how God saved his people: by destroying their enemies.

Part II: Being Formed - Decade II

Our religious life changed a bit when I was nine because my dad had an otherworldly experience, the kind of experience people have eating magic mushrooms, only without the shrooms. He filtered that experience through the lens of a charismatic Christian, meaning he interpreted it as a God encounter and attributed it to the power of the Holy Spirit. Not long after, Dad decided to leave his six-figure job in sales and start his own church. With eight of their friends, my parents started a church that would grow to a congregation of more than 2,000. This is the church I would attend through college and where I would eventually work.

Not a lot changed when we moved churches. We still attended Sunday school and church services every week. God was still good and loving, and we still believed Jesus came to Earth as God in the flesh and died to pay for our sins. Salvation was free to all who believed. Literally free. All you had to do was believe the story. It was our job to make sure everyone knew this love was free! Again, all you had to do was believe the story. *Wait, doesn't that mean I have to do something to get something for free? Then it's not really free, is it?* I struggled with that.

Indoctrination can be relaxing: When you go along with it, you're simply on the right side; you don't have to think for yourself. Essential to its success—and this is whether the indoctrination is coming from home or school or church or country—is that you don't question it. You certainly don't ask questions. Which is how I became someone who, from age nine, held true to evangelical doctrine. The Bible was fact. There was a hell of fire for those who didn't profess with their mouths that Jesus was their personal Lord and savior. There was one way of interpreting scripture, and it was the way we were interpreting it. God created Adam and Eve, not Adam and Steve. Abortion was bad. Capital punishment was good. War was a necessary means to an end, and God was always on the side of the US. Men were head of the household, women a lesser vessel. Getting drunk was bad and having sex outside of the context of marriage was really, really bad. If you just believed, and followed all the rules, life would go better for you.

When I was around eleven years old, my favorite action figure toy and cartoon was He-Man and the Masters of the Universe. I could play with those toys for hours, He-Man conquering Skeletor in Castle Grayskull. I amassed a great He-Man army over a two-year period, scoring new action figures and props every birthday and Christmas. I even used trips to the pediatrician's office as opportunities to acquire new action figures, as my mom always bought my sister and me new toys when we had to get shots. And then there was the daily afternoon cartoon, four o'clock every Monday through Friday. One day my dad asked if he could watch He-Man with me. He wanted to see what it was all about. It's never good when your evangelical dad says he just wants to see what kinds of things you're allowing into your life. I knew what that really meant. And I was, oh, so right.

After the episode, Dad looked at me and said, "You know, Brian, there's really only one master of the universe, and that's Jesus. I think we should pray and think about not watching He-Man anymore, and getting rid of your He-Man toys."

I'm still not sure what went wrong. Maybe we were praying to different gods, because I was certain that whomever I was praying to told me I could keep my toys. But lo and behold, a few days later, Mom and Dad came to my bedroom with a large black garbage bag, and I bid farewell to He-Man and all of his comrades and enemies. And that was it. No more He-Man toys. No more He-Man cartoon-watching afternoons.

One surefire way to ensure you were getting it right was to remove anything that might distract you from Jesus.

I also remember when we lost Mardi Gras. Once a year, people flood the sidewalks and neutral grounds all over the New Orleans metro area as beautiful floats wind their way through the streets and costumed riders throw beads and trinkets to all parade-goers. There are local high school bands, dance teams, and celebrities reigning as kings and queens. And it's not just one parade; the party lasts for weeks. I didn't really know much about Mardi Gras when I was young, except that it was fun. Apparently, though, those parades with names like Iris, Bacchus, and Thoth were named after ancient Roman and Greek gods, and when we unassuming parade-goers lifted our hands upwards toward the heavens while screaming, "Throw me somethin', mister!"—without knowing it, we were raising our hands in worship to pagan gods. So, Mardi Gras became a no-go for our family for about eight years. It wasn't until my junior year of high school that I somehow convinced my parents to allow me to make my way back to Mardi Gras.

I was okay with this God that was handed to me, but whoever this God was, he did seem like an insecure prude, threatened by cartoon characters and beads raining down from drunk dudes on floats.

As I grew older, I began to realize this same God was also threatened by Muslims, Jews, smokers, trick-or-treaters, gays and lesbians, lotto winners, whores, pacifists, and many others. I began to realize this God needed defending. This God's honor was at stake. This God was gravely angered by sin in the world and could have nothing to do with sin, unholiness, imperfection, or anyone who found themselves in these conditions.

I remember being taught as a teenager that God was so disgusted by sin and evil that God couldn't even stand in the presence of sin. Which is why a person must repent, accept the death and punishment of Jesus, hit their knees, beg of God to forgive them for their scumbagedness, and hope for some type of mercy. This understanding of God is especially problematic for teenage boys who like to masturbate because it feels impossible we could ever be accepted by God. Plus, all the kittens we were killing. (There was a running joke when I was in college that every time you jerk off, God kills a kitten). So, we forever repent for masturbating and promise to never do it again. Until tomorrow.

During high school I was required to go to church, and I didn't mind it. We even had a youth group, so I had a handful of friends there, which made it fun. I knew I was on the right side. In 1996, when I was nineteen, during my sophomore year of college, I had what I understood to be an encounter with God. That's the only language I had at the time. It was one of those moments when your soul connects to something deeper and bigger than yourself. We all experience such moments, and not everyone attributes them to God, but we in the evangelical church did—so I did. After that I was all in. So much so that I took a semester off and did a two-month internship at the Anaheim Vineyard Church in Southern California, which at the time was the largest church in our denomination, and where Vineyard churches started. It was our own little Mecca. There and then, I jumped into the deep end. There and then, I developed a passion for God and a heart for people, and I desperately wanted others to experience this love of God. There and then, I felt drawn into pastoral ministry. These things resonated with my soul.

When I returned to New Orleans, I completed a degree in psychology, and then upon my graduation in 1999, I took a job as associate pastor at my dad's church. I was twenty-two years old, young and eager and passionate. I was a sponge, reading anything and everything that could teach me how to win others to the faith. I had no good questions. Even though I had lived very little life, I believed I had studied enough to possess the answers to life's deepest questions. I rode that wave for quite a while.

Part III: The Luckiest Guy on the Planet (Ages 20-28)

The first time I ever laid eyes on Kristy, I was twenty-three. She was sixteen. I don't really remember her from that night because she was Becky's little sister, and I was at their home to pick up Becky for a first date. Becky and I weren't feeling the connection after a few dates, but we seemed to do friendship well; we stayed connected, and over the next year I would see Kristy from time to time.

Late one afternoon while cutting through the Barnes & Noble parking lot, I saw Kristy walking with her mom to their minivan, rolled down my window, and called to her. She bounced over to my car, bubbly, full of life and joy. This was the first time I really *saw* Kristy. Her hair was long and straight and brown and beautiful. Her eyes were a gorgeous green, like looking into an emerald pool. She was the most beautiful girl I had ever seen. I don't know what we talked about that day, but I remember giving her my business card. Maybe I wrote my cell phone number on it. Maybe I somehow thought beautiful seventeen-year-old girls were impressed by twenty-four-year-old pastors. Whatever it was, I was taken by her carefree personality and her beauty.

That was more than twenty-two years ago, so I'm a little fuzzy on the timeline, but in the spring of 2001, we began playing volleyball together at Coconut Beach, a sand volleyball complex. I was in love, but there were two problems: She was seventeen, and she had a boyfriend. I had no choice but to play the long game. Once she graduated from high school and I started driving her to our games, we had about thirty minutes in the car together en route, and then afterward we usually stopped for sno-balls (New Orleans-style shaved ice). During these times alone I would ask questions about her boyfriend, about their relationship, about why she was playing volleyball with me—you know, questions that were intended to help her see who the right guy was for her. But I never said that. I just asked questions. One afternoon she called to say she'd decided to break up with the boyfriend but had no way to get to his house to tell him. I did what any friend would do and offered to drive her there. Sitting outside in my car while she was inside breaking up with her boyfriend still ranks as one of the greatest moments in my life. Once she turned eighteen, we began dating.

Spirituality was much more important to me than it was to Kristy. She'd gone to church most of her life but had somehow avoided indoctrination. Her approach to spirituality and life was simple: Life is to be lived and enjoyed, don't overthink it, and love. This was incredibly attractive to me. We were married eighteen months later, when I was twenty-six and she was nineteen. We had our first son, Micah, in 2004 and became pregnant with our second son, Jonah, in early 2005. As we started our family, I was excited to begin raising our boys in the way of the faith.

Part IV: Hurricanes and Worldviews (Ages 29-32)

On August 29, 2005, Hurricane Katrina barreled down on New Orleans and destroyed the city and much of its outskirts. The brand-new church building we were scheduled to move into the same weekend of the storm sustained a quarter million dollars' worth of damage. We didn't know it at the time, but life and church would never look the same. Hurricane Katrina was a defining moment in my life and for my soul, a turning point. I no longer recognized the ground beneath my feet. Up to this point, my life and career had been devoted to reading books on apologetics, to studying how to win others to Christ, and to teaching others to do the same. But now. Now people were living in FEMA trailers in their front yards for what would turn out to be years as they tried to rebuild their homes and, in many cases, their lives. Suddenly, winning people to Christ didn't seem like the right target; nor did trying to get people "saved" from an eventual postmortem hell. People seemed to be experiencing a hell on earth, and what they really needed was a warm meal or a shoulder to cry on or a hand in gutting their home. Perhaps for the first time ever, it felt like belonging to a church actually mattered; as a community we were able to help people solve real problems.

I was at a crossroads where my choices were either to double down on what I'd been taught, or lay down some of my cards and make the harder choice to allow a new reality to form me, to see what this new terrain could teach me. It was an opportunity to listen and tend to my soul, and I took it. The storm destroyed our home and everything we owned except our little Nissan Sentra. So, Kristy and I got to really start wrestling with questions about God, sovereignty, providence, and much more.

For the next three years we did church differently. Hurricane recovery took precedence over church programs, so we had nothing to invite people to. For the first time ever, we did church outside the church building, spending all our time and energy in the community doing whatever we could to care for others. At the same time, our family continued to grow—because what better way to deal with disaster than having sex and making babies? Our third son, Nathan, was born in 2007, and number four, Lucas, followed in 2008. We were our own traveling preschool with four boys under the age of five.

As my family expanded, so did my world. I developed a desire to travel as part of missionary work, which led me to Africa, Mexico, and even on a pilgrimage to Israel and the Palestinian territory. Again I felt the ground beneath my feet shifting. I met Jews and Muslims, the poorest of the poor in Mexico, and the people of Zambia, Eritrea, Botswana, and Ethiopia. During this post-Katrina time of imposed transition, I was also introduced to some new authors who began to open my mind and challenge some of my tightly held beliefs, authors who painted a more beautiful picture of the Christian religion than what I'd been taught. Their Christianity elevated beauty, inclusion, grace, and love, and it devalued judgmentalism and black-and-white thinking. These authors put language to feelings I'd been experiencing for a number of years in my soul.

Even though my ideas about human ontology were spreading out, and the way I'd been taught to read and interpret the scriptures was being challenged, at the time I didn't consider my changing worldview to be a crisis of faith. It felt more like an expansion. It felt like I was waking up. For the first time ever, the way of Jesus actually looked like some kind of good news. My soul was catching on fire, and I was beginning to ask good questions again. Baby steps.

Part V: The Perfect Storm (Ages 33-38)

By age thirty-three, I had a bit more life under my belt. I'd been married for seven years. We had four children and were in the process of adopting our daughter from Ethiopia. I'd learned enough theology to be asking bigger questions. For example, my oldest son was nearly seven, the age when I was baptized and "saved." Abandoning the belief that my seven-year-olds would need to be forgiven their sins to avoid being cast away by God was an early sign of my realizing I'd been traveling down the wrong road. After all, I was already a more loving and compassionate and forgiving father than the God I was raised to know.

More questions from this time—or, rather, answers: It was clear to me now that everything does not happen for a reason. Also, if God is the one dishing out life, then God absolutely *does* give us more than we can handle. And if God is good and knows the future, and has all power and doesn't use that power to prevent injustice—nope, that wasn't going to work for me anymore. We taught people that God cares so deeply about every part of your life that asking for a good parking spot at the mall, or nice weather for your kid's birthday party, was a valid use of prayer. So, we worshiped a God that wanted to help us get a good parking spot but didn't feel compelled to insert himself during the Holocaust? Nope, that no longer worked for me either.

In a perfect storm kind of scenario, right as I was coming to these conclusions, I was presented with a job promotion, an event that pushed me down the greatest and scariest path of my soul journey to that point. It happened like this: One day I took my dad to the hospital for a medical procedure that required anesthesia. I was able to sit with him in the recovery area after the procedure, as he came to. When he was still loopy from the meds, he told me a hundred times that he loved me and was proud of me. He also told me that he and his church's board had put into writing that I would be my dad's successor. I was the one they intended to train and develop into the next lead pastor of this church of what was then 1,400 people, with a five-year transition plan to begin immediately. I instantaneously felt a heavy weight descend, and an internal dialogue began.

Is this what I want? Am I up for this? Do we need to pray about it? Holy shit, this is so cool. I can't do this. I was made for this. I don't want to do this.

My soul got the final word: I didn't want this. But I wanted to want it, so I tried. After some fits and starts, prayers for peace and clarity, and ignoring my soul's answer, I was finally settled into the position after about a year. I can't say whether the depression I began to experience during this time arose from not listening to my soul, or whether I didn't listen to my soul because depression had come calling. Maybe the two aren't even related. What I can say is that the depression didn't leave once I committed to the job. It would come and go on its own time for many years. Sometimes it would hover for a few hours, and sometimes it would stick around for a few months. I told myself I was just scared and nervous. A fear to fight through. A closed door I needed to kick down. Par for the course.

In hindsight, and after much therapy and reflection, I see I was afraid of letting down my dad, our staff, and our congregation. I felt stuck. My soul tried to speak, and I silenced it. Little by little my soul got the picture. It became increasingly shy and timid, hiding away in the corner. My soul tried so hard, but it finally went dormant, waiting for me to pay attention to it. Waiting to be invited into the conversation.

I had life and God and purpose and love all figured out. Until I didn't. And so, in my first six years of pastoring I only read books and listened to people who already agreed with how I believed. (I actually did read some books that disagreed with what I was teaching, but only so I could adequately teach against them.) They reassured me how right I was. But it didn't work. I prayed for our God to heal sick people who never got healed. I did funerals for babies born dead and for cops killed in the line of duty, leaving behind wives and small children. I held the hands of rape victims. I stood at the bedside with men and women as they said good-bye to the one person they loved most in the world. I saw families destroyed when someone in the family came out as gay against their religious beliefs. I kept at it, but this God wasn't working for me. And my soul knew it.

My conscious mind didn't consider leaving the family church, but my questions were gaining momentum. I decided to channel that energy into creating a one-year class to explore with a small group of people what a truly Jesus-like life would look like. After all, Jesus never said, "Worship me"; he just said, "Follow me and the way I live." To develop the class, I needed to read and study outside my wheelhouse. I easily read sixty books in preparation. The curriculum not only encouraged questions; it had questions built into it. I stayed in the Christian lane but began to learn about nonevangelical Christians who interpreted the scriptures in radically different ways from what I'd been taught. It was scary and invigorating, and I stumbled upon messages and ways of doing religion I could get behind. There were many alternative ways of understanding the Jesus story that resonated deeply with my soul.

One example is how I'd been taught that Jesus died on the cross because God demanded a blood sacrifice for sin; Jesus died on the cross to save us humans; God was too holy to allow sin and sinners in his presence, a price had to be paid, and God was willing to let his one and only sinless son be tortured and murdered instead of us. This story makes God out to be one of the most maniacal, abusive dads of all time, and the more I read, the less the story lined up with the image of God that Jesus's teachings seemed to convey. Once I realized there were other ways of understanding Jesus's death, I picked one that sat a little better with me: A man named Jesus actually died and then came back from the dead to overcome the power of evil and death, thus allowing all of creation to live free, out from under the power of evil. This is an overly simplistic explanation of a very complex theological question, but you get the gist. The point being, I encountered new ways of thinking that I could teach with integrity. I invested in Jesus at a deeper level, and it felt right and good.

Theology was something I didn't just absorb and assimilate anymore, but something I wrestled with. Really wrestled with. I wrestled with questions outside the Jesus story, like how to reconcile the God of the Old Testament and the God of the New Testament—a difference that seemed irreconcilable. I then spent a year or so diving into same-sex relationships, trying to figure out why the Christian tradition considered it sin. And I just kept going with the questions. I taught the course for five years as I continued to study and improve it.

Once I decided everything was up for questioning, I went straight for the jugular and one of the Christian precepts that never jibed with me. Hell. It never made sense. Again, new-to-me writings helped me find my own way through the maze of reconciling a loving God and such a gruesome eternal destiny for nonbelievers. I moved through many stages of belief, finally giving up on hell altogether, and maybe heaven too.

I just reread that last paragraph and must say I've made the journey I undertook sound like a systematic, efficient, easy, quick process of challenging firmly held, intensely ingrained beliefs. It was not any of that. This took years of wrestling both internally and externally.

Here's an important thing to know about beginning to question deeply held truths and unexamined dogma: It has the potential to drive you mad. You'll likely experience anxiety and unsettled nerves. I was really in it. By the time I was thirty-six, it did indeed feel like a crisis of faith. I didn't journey and change my beliefs in a vacuum. I took eight trusted companions, including my dad, with me. I had no choice but to lay all my cards on the table. About everything. No holds barred. That time in my life was difficult, scary, exciting, and insanely challenging and exhausting. But we were safe with each other and loved one another as brothers and sisters. We haven't all landed in the same place, but we continue to wrestle and journey together to this day.

At this point, the gates were flung wide open. In coming to understand the Bible as a book of myths and stories about people wrestling with God and interpreting their own lives with God, I was able to appreciate it more. I could get on board with it. As I moved further down the path, my soul felt like it was coming to life. Or maybe like I was finally listening to it.

My spiritual practice narrowed in on what kind of person I wanted to be. I kept coming back to Jesus's saying, essentially, "If you want to live a life of inner peace and a life of mercy and love and grace, a life free, then follow my lead." The teachings and life of Jesus felt like a way to live and experience my humanity while living. This wasn't about worshiping Jesus. Just following. I didn't need the threat of hell to make me want to live a Jesus-like life.

When you take worship out of the equation and just focus on following, a lot of the things evangelical Christians argue against look ridiculous. I mean, following Jesus means following a guy who made weddings more fun, a guy who always had a seat at his table for anyone, a guy who was comfortable in his own skin, a guy who could see the dangers and pitfalls in how people were living and encourage them to change their minds about their choices. This was a guy who was murdered, came back to life, found his murderers, and said, "All is good. I forgive you." This is a guy who was accused of being a glutton and a drunk. I started wondering, *Why aren't more of Jesus's followers being accused of being gluttons and drunks? Maybe we're doing it wrong.* The only people Jesus didn't like being around were the rule makers and enforcers, and the exclusionists.

As right and good as the conclusions felt in my soul, all this journeying took a toll on my mental health. I was changing my mind about truths that had been foundational in my life for decades, and it was scary. In my experience, it's pretty common to suffer great anxiety before deep peace anytime you transition away from long-held, deeply ingrained beliefs.

By the fall of 2014, when I was thirty-eight, I had reached a crossroads: I either needed to get out of pastoring altogether, or I needed to find a place where I could practice my faith differently. My dad's church (by now it was mine too) was making huge strides in the same direction I was going, but it wasn't moving quickly enough for me. And I didn't feel up to the task of leading a huge, well-established church through new theological and doctrinal ideas. It felt too massive for me, and I didn't want to do it. Most importantly, I finally was ready to follow my soul and what my soul had started whispering five years earlier.

Part VI: A New Beginning (Ages 39-43)

Kristy and I always felt we belonged in the city. We dreamed of relocating from the suburbs once our kids were grown and out of the house. But the sea change in my belief system and my desire to pastor differently were the push we needed to make the move now, both to a home in the city and to the small church we started.

Midcity Church was a small, completely inclusive group more interested in how we ourselves lived than proselytizing to others. Some of our fellow founders came from my dad's church, either because they had a similar desire to join a new faith community, or because they lived in the city and were interested in what we were trying to do. We had two goals: (1) to learn to love each other, and (2) to love our community in whatever ways we could. And we did it. For five years we were a staple in our community. About forty strong, aged two to seventy-eight, we gathered on Saturday evenings to worship together. We built our community around the communion table, literally—we sat in a circle around our communion table, which we assembled each week anew from cinder blocks and rugged fence boards. The blocks and boards represented the raw materials that made up our lives, and the table was the place where we could lay all our differences aside and break bread together. Each week someone spoke about the ways of Jesus and how we might follow Jesus's lead in the ways of love. We then opened the floor for conversation and concluded our time by sharing communion. Everyone was welcome to partake. We also got together twice a week to eat and drink, and in so doing learn how to tend to our souls and how to be present here and now.

It was incredible. Those of us who stuck it out learned together how to live in harmony. How to extend grace. How to forgive. How to love. We learned how to work through conflict. We were committed to each other and to doing our best to live the way Jesus lived. So much so that some wondered if we were gluttons and drunks. We practiced a Christianity that looked as close to Jesus as I'd ever seen. We comprised eight different ethnicities. Straight people. Gay people. Six figures and those who couldn't pay the rent. Democrats and Republicans. Addicts. Recovering addicts. We had at least one of every kind, and we agreed together that Jesus's way seemed good to us, and we pursued it together without judgment. Without the baggage of superfluous rules and the weight of getting it right.

As beautiful as it was to start and grow that church, I wearied of explaining to people, "Yes, I'm a Christian, but not that kind." Beyond that, I liked the Jesus path, but my mind was continuing to expand, and I no longer saw Jesus's way as the only way to find true joy and happiness and contentment in life. Certainly it was one way, but not the only way. The more I studied and got real with my soul, the surer I became that Jesus's one goal had been to show people what a life could look like if a person stayed true to their internal compass. Their soul. I was a pastor in the Christian tradition, so my soul growth was beginning to feel uncomfortable. And a bit like we were engaging in multi-level marketing. Pick us. We're the Christians who have figured it out. I was reaching a spiritual place that was unfigureoutable, and I wanted to keep going in that direction.

Then it happened. Four years into pastoring this small group, at the age of forty-three, I was diagnosed with ALS. A terminal disease, and the doctor telling me I wouldn't make it to my forty-eighth birthday. Now this is where theology comes into play for real, theology being the way someone thinks God and/or the universe plays the game of life. People would ask me, "Are you mad at God?" But I hadn't thought God was all-knowing or all-powerful for years. I figured God found out I had ALS at the precise moment when Dr. Edwards looked at Kristy and me and said, "I'm so sorry. You have ALS." God also got sucker-punched. God was too busy saying, "Fuuuuck!" to also get blamed. That would be unfair. So, no, I'm not mad at God.

Part VII: Leaving My Chucks

I didn't feel like doing much with the church after my diagnosis. We kept it going for one more year, mostly because Covid was in full force. People needed it. We gathered over Zoom once a week, concentrating only on the Jesus stories. I knew early on, though, that it wasn't going to work for me. I still loved the stories, but they were just stories to me at this point. All that mattered to me was the way Jesus had lived. A life of peace, love, and presence. I'd finally stripped it down, all the way down.

Because we loved the story it tells of a soul on a journey, we would sing U2's song "I Still Haven't Found What I'm Looking For" in church. We would hang on the last verse, so powerful with its

ON JOURNEY

imagery of loosened chains and a cross of shame, and then preach messages about how you can only find true hope and love in God. *See everyone! This is it. This is where you finally find what you've been looking for. It's all found in the Jesus story. This is the secret to a beautiful life. Not easy but a whole and beautiful life.* This is how our conversations and preachings would go. And I still loved it. I so wanted this to be it.

And then the next line after that powerful verse is the famous chorus, "But I still haven't found what I'm looking for."

Which is how I've always felt too. I'd done everything I could think of to feel whole, and I'd gotten so close I could taste it. I'd spent my entire life searching for that one piece to complete the puzzle. For a while that piece was Jesus. I liked Jesus, and I liked my new understanding of the Jesus story: how Jesus had everything to do with being awake and present to this life, but many tenets of the faith I could no longer adhere to. And what I finally realized is that I no longer need any of these stories to be true.

I want to repeat that because this is where the gold is: I no longer needed it to be true.

For years I'd needed it to all be true. It was my security blanket. It served as my compass. But ultimately the Jesus journey was my way to finding and caring for, and eventually trusting, my own soul. I was and am a believer that the world and life are full of love and magic for those who have eyes to see it. My journey with Jesus opened my eyes to a whole new world, but I now understand Jesus wasn't the point. Whatever/whomever Jesus was pointing to was the point.

The ground beneath my feet had once again shifted. Only this time did I realize how whatever had gotten me to this point in life was not going to take me on the next, possibly final, leg of my journey. I was entering the unknowable, the place of unwritten stories, and it would be up to me to find a way through. My Converse had served me well. These Converse had been good to me. They had fit me perfectly. I loved these shoes. They were worn and torn in the best ways. They had stuck with me through it all, from an ambitious little fundamentalist who could defeat any critic with a solid answer from God's perfect word, the Bible—gun-loving, American flag-waving, anti-abortion, pro-war, pro-capital punishment, and definitely Adam and Eve, no Steve—to the person I am today. Which is, well, none of those things.

I'd laced up these Converse for the first time at age nineteen, when I chose to follow Jesus, and wore them every day since. I was wearing them in Anaheim. I was wearing them the day I became a pastor. I was wearing them on 9/11, during Hurricane Katrina, when I got married, when all five kids came home. They were with me when life started kicking the shit out of me. When my whole world went black, and hopelessness was the deep end of the ocean, and I was desperately trying not to drown. On the day I betrayed a dear friend, and on days when friends left me. They saw me through major paradigm shifts. They never failed me. Always waiting to be laced up for a new day of surprises. Come hell or high water.

These Converse weren't just Converse; they were my companions, and they represented trust, loyalty, service, and friendship.

But it was time. Christianity took me as far as it could. It made me the person I was, and now it felt too small to take me where I needed to go next. Where I was being invited was bigger and more mysterious. So, with gratitude in my heart, and tears in my eyes, I slowly unlaced my Converse for the last time.

It was time to move onward, forward* without them.

So, I left my Converse behind.

In that one moment of surrender, as I placed my Chuck Taylors on the altar that is my life, it felt as if I were embarking on a new and sacred journey. My eyes were opened to a whole new world. I felt awake and alive and more connected. Taking all that was good and beautiful and lovely from the beginning of the journey and building on it.

Yes, I have ALS. And yet today, my soul is whole. I feel fully connected to myself, to others, to creation. I experience the world and everything in it as sacred. I live with a soul fully alive and connected. I'm connected to the Oneness. My soul is at rest, and I am free. I have found what I was looking for.

Life is a beautiful clusterfuck and love is here.
Onward. Forward.*
love.

CHAPTER 3

ON ONENESS

> *"Are you there God, it's me,
> Margaret's little boy,
> long-time listener, first-time caller."*
> —Coach Beard*

My initial thought was to name this chapter "On God" and then leave the next fourteen pages blank. How are finite creatures to talk about the infinite? It would be like me trying to write a chapter on quantum physics or brain surgery. However, people have been trying to write about the infinite for thousands and thousands of years. And no one knows for sure, so they write down their thoughts and musings based on their own experience. And that's now what I shall attempt.

As soon as Fantine opened her mouth and began to sing "I Dreamed a Dream" in a performance of Les Misérables at the Saenger Theatre in New Orleans, I was teleported to a different space where all of life felt connected. The same thing happened the first time I saw the documentary *Gleason*, as I sat in the theater for twenty minutes after the credits rolled, weeping.

I remember hiking the Grand Canyon on a snowy day in late December with my family and knowing in my bones we were part of something bigger than ourselves. I felt it at the christening of my friend's new baby boy. I felt it at a U2 concert in Houston as 40,000 of us sang "I Still Haven't Found What I'm Looking For" in unison. I felt it when I had the honor of officiating my best friend's wedding. I felt it when another friend invited me to a small chapel for midnight prayers on Christmas Eve, only five of us there sitting in the sacred silence. I felt it when I saw Susan Boyle's audition for *Britain's Got Talent*. I felt it when the Avett Brothers closed their show with "No Hard Feelings." I felt it when I had the opportunity to sit with and talk to Alanis Morissette. I feel it when I make love to my wife.

And I felt it in February 2010 when the New Orleans Saints recovered the onside kick and Tracey Porter picked off Peyton Manning and the Saints won the Superbowl. That might be the closest I've ever felt to what the world's potential could be, filled with joy and goodness, laughter and love. What a possible heaven might be like. I don't understand cities that riot when their teams win, turning over cars and burning the town down. In New Orleans, we danced in the streets, literally for weeks. Violent crimes went down, and there were no murders for days—a sure sign of something miraculous happening here. Music filled the streets, and you didn't meet any strangers, only other Who Dats.

I could go on. We've all felt it at some point. A connectedness that transcends us as individuals. A moment when we realize we're part of something. Something bigger than ourselves.

I've always loved questions, and I wrestled with questions about the Christian tradition even as I served as a pastor for twenty-two years, my entire career. By the time I was diagnosed with ALS in 2020, my theology had already evolved. I was a Christian Universalist, meaning I no longer believed in hell; I believed all of humanity would be welcomed into a postmortem paradise, or heaven, through Jesus. I believed homosexuality was a beautiful and acceptable expression of love. I no longer believed people were born inherently bad. I didn't think Jesus had tried to save people from a postmortem hell—he'd tried to help people live their one life, present and free and full of love. I'd also come to a place of not believing God was all-powerful or all-knowing.

These aren't mainstream teachings on the Christian God. Most Christians would consider them heretical, actually, but I suggest that's only because they have God in a box. Boxing God in isn't limited to the Christian tradition. All religions do it. Religions exist because, as a species, we're afraid of mystery and uncertainty and the unknown. We can't control life, which is, honestly, scary AF, so we construct gods that have control. Some people choose to believe that life is already mapped out for each of us. Everything happens for a reason, and all things unfold just as they should. Some even believe the gods know everything that's going to happen.

I get it. I camped out here for part of my life, which I think gives me license to call it as I see it. This belief system of an all-knowing, all-powerful God alleviates the burden of taking ownership of our own lives. It's comforting, and we might feel safer, to believe everything is predetermined. I've been there, and if you're currently camping out with this belief and it's working for you, then feel free to stay put. I am, however, still going to call it what it is: control.

Our incessant need for control is like a cancer in our bodies that kills us slowly. Our need for control occupies real estate in our minds and is never content, often causing us to be paralyzed with fear. Control is an illusion that allows us to rest, trusting in a God who's pulling the strings. We pray to this God for our children's protection when we drop them off at school. We pray for a safe flight when we travel. We pray for our loved ones' good health, and we pray for financial success in our business ventures. And everything is great and we feel comfortable in our lives because God is in control and we can trust God.

Until a gunman walks into our child's school and blows away twenty children and four teachers, including our sweet seven-year-old, Ophelia. Or our loved one's plane goes down, or our child is killed by a drunk driver. Now what do we do? Many people double down. *Well, God's plans are bigger than our understanding.* Or, *God is in the business of working all things together for good for those who love him.* Or, *God knew before the foundations of the earth this would happen, so there is a reason.* Doubling down like this is a coping mechanism. Nothing more.

It's tempting to want every victory to be a blessing from God, and every defeat, every tragedy, every nightmare to be known ahead of time by God—there's solace in believing God is the reason for everything. But what kind of God is that, besides a cruel, vindictive God who keeps us on a string like a marionette? Besides that, this is exactly what makes God *not* God: when we can figure God out.

For the entire first year after my diagnosis, I spent almost every night on my front porch, by myself. I didn't read one book or listen to one podcast. No TED talks or YouTube videos. Nothing. No input. I thought. And I meditated. And I prayed. And I thought. And I pondered. And I prayed. And I meditated. And I thought. And I sifted through more than a quarter century of input, throwing everything I had read, been taught, and learned against the wall, determined to only keep what stuck. And honestly, not much stuck. On countless nights I found myself conversing with the God I'd constructed over the course of my life and wondering how to move forward together. I flirted with atheism and agnosticism but didn't really connect with either. Agnosticism looked like a decent path, and if it turns out there's nothing after this and no greater being, I'm fine with that. But at around the six-month mark, something happened. Each night, as the tug-of-war on my porch waged on, I began to sense presence with me. I knew I wasn't alone. And as the year progressed, I felt a connection to something bigger and more beautiful and better and more loving than even the pretty good God I had constructed.

I recall saying out loud, "Who are you?" And even asking, "What do I call you?" and "What is your name?" I felt like Moses at the burning bush asking this being he'd never experienced before, "So, when I walk into Egypt and tell the most powerful man in the world, Pharaoh, to let his millions of slaves go, who should I tell him sent me? Seriously, though, what is your name?"

To which he received the answer, "I am that I am."

I'm sure Moses felt incredibly confident with such a ridiculous name backing him up. The point is that Moses, who was probably under the influence of magic mushrooms at the time (I mean, I wasn't there, but I have to imagine it was a real possibility), had to ask this thing or being or God what its name was. Why? Because he'd never encountered anything like it. So was true with me. Sitting alone on my front porch, sometimes into the early morning hours, I began to encounter something I'd not encountered before. And this. This was bigger than what I'd been calling God. What I was encountering on my porch made what I'd been calling God seem tiny. Not insignificant, but still very, very small.

It got deep. For the first time, I recognized a singular thread weaving its way through every human being, every squirrel, every oak tree and river and mountain and valley and star and solar system, in a way that connects us all. Even the word God was suddenly too small. More pressingly, the name God carried with it too much negative baggage. I spent many a night asking it, *What do I call you?*

I landed on Oneness because Oneness seems to encompass the experience of feeling everything is connected and interdependent. When I stumbled upon Alanis Morissette's 2020 album, *Such Pretty Forks in the Road* and heard her refer to the Oneness in the song "Ablaze," that confirmed my answer. (Perhaps more interesting, Alanis played God in the 1999 movie *Dogma*. Isn't it ironic? Don't you think?)

Of course, I don't really think it matters what I call it. I'm cool with its remaining nameless. However, I don't like referring to it as "whatever this thing is that holds everything together" in conversation. It's such a clunky mouthful. So, it's Oneness or Allness, which I also took from Alanis.

Oneness is what holds everything together. The Oneness has only one job description, and that's love. Binding universes and solar systems and human hearts together in love. Oneness isn't in the business of controlling lives or pulling the strings like a master puppeteer. The Oneness isn't interested in running the show, or even intervening. At the same time, the Oneness isn't aloof and disconnected. It's not so much a being to be worshiped as an essence to be lived into, for Oneness is the constant in life, the ground of our being, drawing all of creation into deeper relationship and love. Those who have eyes to see and a soul to experience will recognize that the Oneness is the water we swim in and the air we breathe.

If I'm wrong about this and the Christian tradition is correct, I'm confident Jesus, as I understand him, will still have a seat at his table for me. I'll probably be sitting in the back next to Judas, but at least we'll have plenty of stories to share over a good bottle of bourbon. It's a great idea to find someone to model your own life after. The Dalai Lama, Mr. Magorium, the Buddha, your sweet grandmother, Jesus, Ted Lasso. If you pick Jesus, don't get bogged down in the weeds. Don't argue about stupid stuff.

Speaking of Jesus, he called it Abba or Father. Moses called it I Am. Jews call it Yahweh. Christians call it God. Muslims call it Allah. Hindus call it Brahman. We're all looking for that one thing that binds us together. That one thread that weaves itself through all of creation. And for some bizarre reason we're intent on fighting one another, even killing, over which of us is more right. Damn, it's exhausting. It wore me out. We're all looking for the same thing, that much was clear. So, I tapped out of the religion game, and I'm devoting the rest of my life to learning how to love well. We are all born with this capacity to love. Contrary to what I learned from a young age, I believe our soul, our very essence, is good and pure from the moment we arrive on the planet. Our job is to learn to nurture it and follow it.

On the off chance they find a cure and reversal of this disease, I won't return to pastoring or going to a church. Instead, I'll go back to school, get a degree in physical therapy, and devote the rest of my life to giving away hope.

I'll also run a side business where I invite people to sit on my front porch to explore the depths of soul together. Mostly they'll talk, I'll listen, and then I'll ask them one or two questions until we find ourselves in a whole new realm of existence and connection to each other and the Oneness.

Most importantly, I'll work only as much as I need to contribute to supporting our family with Kristy, who herself has a great many ways of supporting us. To know Kristy is to want to be around Kristy, so people just hire her, if for no other reason than her presence. If you don't know Kristy this way, then unfortunately she probably doesn't like you. Or maybe you've just had trouble breaking through her resting bitch face, RBF. One day early in our marriage, probably around day four, I asked her what was wrong.

"Nothing!" she replied. "Stop asking me that. This is just my normal."

Ah. Duly noted. In my defense, we chose not to live or sleep together before we got married, so I had a lot of new stuff coming at me all at once.

I also sometimes suffer from RBF, and as luck would have it, I will live the rest of my life wearing just one face, but we're calling this Resting Brian Face. It turns out my mom was right: "If you keep making that face, then your face is going to get stuck like that." Oof.

The point being, we would make what we needed, and only what we needed, and spend the rest of our time being together and with our kids and with our neighbors and friends, investing all we have into presence and love. Telling our lives how we are going to spend them, and not letting work or chaos or busyness or other people tell us how to spend our lives.

I know this chapter is supposed to be about Oneness. Stick with me, it's all connected. My encouragement is to go after love at all costs. You won't be disappointed. Develop your inner life. Nurture it. Care for it. And take time to develop the eyes of your soul to recognize and experience the Oneness in every moment of every day. (See? There it is.) For there's no greater treasure in any life than being fully here for it. What good is it to gain the whole world—money and wealth, certainty and control—but lose your life, your soul? The carrot on the stick will always be there, but there's a better way. It's going to cost you everything. Complete surrender. To life. To control. To love. This is the road less traveled. This is the road to life. This is the road to love. This is the road to Oneness. And here's the thing about surrender: If none of what I feel is true, if this life is it, and there's no Oneness or afterlife or anything, I'm okay with that. It doesn't change anything about how I invest this life.

More encouragement. Wherever you find yourself today, keep going. One foot in front of the other. Just pay attention. Try opening your eyes to the Oneness you're a part of and integral to. You're living it, right now, in this moment, and this is the only moment you can experience it. By which I mean, this moment is the only moment we're guaranteed. This is it. If you're spending the present moment worrying about your flight tomorrow, you're missing out on experiencing the Oneness right now. The flight will happen, or not, in spite of your worry, so why not choose the Oneness? The world is full of life and love and magic for those who have eyes to see. Everything is alive with spirit and soul. We're integrally connected as interdividuals. There's no me without you. Everything is sacred and holy.

Whether you're following Abraham's lead or Gandhi's or Jesus's or Muhammad's or your grandmother's, just make sure you're growing in the way of love. What does it mean to grow in love? You feel your soul and your life expanding. If instead you feel yourself becoming smaller, then you're going the wrong way. Change your mind and change directions. You're invited to be here.

When we learn to recognize and live every second of life fully present to the moment, whimsically dancing with the Oneness and

ON ONENESS

life—we'll sell everything for this. So, I've not given up on spirituality. I submit I'm more enmeshed in the sacred than ever in my life before. The world is alive and ablaze. I now see it *all* as spiritual, *all* as sacred. Everything is sacred. Every. Thing. Is. Sacred. Oneness.

Life is a beautiful clusterfuck and love is here. Onward. Forward.*
love.

CHAPTER 4

ON SOUL

*"Explore the world.
More importantly, explore yourself."*
—Deborah Welton*

Our family has had the opportunity to travel a bit, and on some of my favorite trips—to the Smoky Mountains, the Rockies, the Grand Canyon, and others—we've wound up in caves. Nowadays, caves are built out with elevators for transporting tourists hundreds of feet below the earth's surface, and lighted pathways to aid in navigating the cold, wet, underground mazes. I'm intrigued by the stalagmites and stalactites, the dampness of the caves, and most of all, the mystery of them. I like to imagine the people who first found the caves, with their pickaxes and candles. I imagine their adrenaline, their uncertainty, their fear, their excitement. I imagine they awoke each morning with joy for what exploration and discovery the day would bring, and I imagine they hoped they wouldn't die in the process.

Just as caves ask to be explored, so too do our inner lives, our souls. Soul can be a confusing concept. Is soul the same as spirit? Is soul limited to humans? Does soul only reside in animate objects? Does soul last forever? What *is* soul?

When I speak of soul, I speak of essence. The truest, most raw and genuine part of our being. Our North Star. Our compass. Our true self.

When I speak of soul, I speak of something malleable. Soul can be formed and shaped. Soul can expand and grow.

When I speak of soul, I speak of something good and trustworthy.

When I speak of soul, I speak of something that requires attention and care. For, soul can be bruised and cut and fractured. It can shrink and hide away. Therefore, soul must be acknowledged and tended to. Soul needs love in all its wholeness and brokenness.

When I speak of soul, I speak of our gift to the world.

When I speak of soul, I speak of connection. Those who understand and accept and love their truest self, their soul, will always recognize others on the journey. Those who know their soul walk with a quiet confidence; they radiate love; and they walk humbly, for in coming to know their soul they've necessarily faced the ugliest parts of themselves. They've seen the best and worst of themselves, and they understand they stand superior to no one. From this moment on, I like to say, they walk with a limp. The greatest example I've witnessed of people accepting all of themselves and thereby getting in touch with their soul is my friends in Alcoholics Anonymous (AA). These men and women are some of the bravest and most vulnerable people I've met. One of my dear friends—I'll call him Manny—has been sober for almost twenty-five years. During his days as an alcoholic, he lived under bridges, was heavily addicted to drugs, and stole from family and friends and strangers to support his addiction. He spent years in and out of jail. Today Manny is one of the most gentle, kind, loving people I know. He passes judgment on no one, as he knows what he himself is capable of. Manny walks with a limp, which is a gift to all who know him.

I don't differentiate between soul and spirit and personhood. Call it what you want. Essence. Spirit. Heart. Consciousness. Gut. I call it soul.

We were created, and driven, to live from soul. That's the whole purpose of religion, yoga, meditation, mindfulness: It's all trying to teach us how to know our true self and live from that place. Unfortunately, most of these disciplines add their own baggage to our journey, especially religion. There are no bad souls, just bad stewards. And bad stewards often steward poorly for reasons beyond their control, including, as I once heard Alanis Morissette say, "History, genetics, trauma, neurological susceptibility, culture ... so many aspects of what blocks or allows flow to these embodied souls."

Upon my ALS diagnosis, I was immediately called to deeper exploration of my inner life. My soul. I'd already spent roughly a decade consciously nurturing my soul, beginning in 2009 when a depression descended and I began asking deeper questions. A couple of years later, I stumbled upon the ancient practice of spiritual direction, or soul care. It had a name, and I began to practice it intentionally. Just as I would go to the gym and run to take care of my physical body, or read and play Sudoku to keep my mind sharp, I began to take greater care of my soul through practices like sitting alone in silence, spending time with myself, and reflecting on my inner life. In addition, I went back to school for two years to learn how to sojourn with others on their journeys inward. I suppose in some ways this was like pastoring, although my role in the co-journeying was to listen, ask questions, and allow people to draw their own conclusions—versus a pastor's typical role of leading people to predetermined conclusions.

Then, in late 2014 and early 2015, the depression hit bottom. I was in a pit of despair and suicidal. That time led me deep into the cave and crevices of my life. I had previously investigated many dark spaces within myself, but I had never gone this deep, where it was this dark and dangerous and frightening. I made it to the bottom of my life. My cave. My soul.

In hindsight, that extended era of soul exploration positioned me for the precise moment of my diagnosis. I had already stared death by suicide in the face by the time doctors told me I had two to five years left to live. I had some new exploring to do, but it was familiar terrain. This time, though, I faced a reality beyond my control: a very difficult life of losses, starting with losing the ability to move. Then, I would lose my ability to eat, speak, and breathe, all of which would inevitably lead to death. I knew what to do. I grabbed my pickaxe and my flashlight and got back to work, first by asking (and answering) questions. *How will I tell my kids? How will I navigate needing a cane to walk? What about not being able to coach my kids anymore, or play with them? What will happen when I can't walk anymore? Or eat? Or speak? What will happen to Kristy and me? Who am I now? How will our family survive now that I can't work? What's my purpose? If I could be dead in two years, how should I spend my time? What's important?* These questions got me even closer to my soul, my essence.

Many of us live disconnected from our souls. We don't allow our souls into the driver's seat. Instead, we allow the external circumstances of our lives dictate who we are. This is missing the point. Our soul knows who we are and what we're for. Best to listen to our souls speaking, allow them to guide our lives.

How, though? How do we make space for our souls to speak, and how do we learn to connect and listen to them?

I hesitate to offer a prescription; it's such personal work. But I can say the greatest way to care for the soul is simple: Pay attention. All the time. During the ordinary and the mundane. I remember complaining about doing chores when I was sixteen years old, specifically about having to wash my clothes, and my mom's saying, "Brian, it is in the ordinary, and only the ordinary, that you can truly experience your life." The reason being that our lives are almost wholly ordinary. Occasionally, we have extraordinary moments, but mostly our lives are lived out at the grocery store, in the carpool line, at work, at the gym, at the ballpark, on our sofas.

Unfortunately, we live in a society that values production and consumption, neither of which is conducive to soul care. In his book, *Care of the Soul: A Guide for Cultivating Depth and Sacredness in Everyday*

Life, Thomas Moore writes, "Soul cannot thrive in a fast-paced life because being affected, taking things in and chewing on them, requires time." In order to truly care for our souls, we must create space and pay attention, especially during ordinary, mundane moments. The ordinary is sacred, even doing the laundry. And as with Oneness, you can only experience your soul in this moment now. I know not whether we're eternal beings (I do suspect we are), so I spend little time thinking about what's coming next. I practice being present to the moment I'm in and not thinking about tomorrow, let alone eternity.

Another nonprescription prescription worth noting: We cannot get to know ourselves or our souls by sitting in a counselor's office for one hour a month. Soul discovery takes real time. Even so, counseling is of utmost importance. I've spent hours and hours in counselors' offices and truly believe everyone should be in counseling. So much so that Kristy and I set aside money for future counseling for our kids so someone can one day help them sort through any damage we unintentionally caused.

The soul must be invited out of hiding. As I previously mentioned, the soul is timid. Most of us spend the first part of our lives pushing our soul into hiding, driven by ego and productivity, and money or fame or lust—qualities that lead us further and further from our true selves. Our souls learn to be quiet. The soul only comes out of hiding when it feels safe, when conditions are quiet and loving.

Here's another nonprescription prescription by way of a story. I once read about a rabbi named Zusya. As an old man, Rabbi Zusya said, "In the coming world, they will not ask me: 'Why were you not Moses?' They will ask me: 'Why were you not Zusya?'"

This is it. Who are you? Your soul will not misguide you. It will lead you to your life.

I don't know all the answers, but I'm pretty sure about this one: Soul is something we all share. All of humankind and all of creation.

From trees and rivers, to squirrels and dogs, to buildings and music. Bridges and benches and beats have soul. Have you ever stepped into an old building and felt as though the walls were speaking its history? Or perhaps you've gazed upon a piece of art that seemed to communicate with you. That's what it's like to experience soul. For, soul is essence. Soul is presence. Soul is intangibly tangible, and soul is experienced by those who have eyes to see, ears to hear, hearts to feel.

In December 2019, our family took a trip to Arizona. We spent days hiking in Sedona, and then went north to the Grand Canyon, where we hiked in the snowy winter. The Grand Canyon is a sight to behold in all its glory and majesty and beauty. I was taken there by the ravens who glided effortlessly through the canyon, seemingly without worries. I distinctly remember imagining how magnificent it must feel to have only one purpose—enjoyment. The ravens seemed to be living in alignment with soul, true to their essence.

We get to choose. We all get to choose. Some of us choose to do the radical hard work of knowing ourselves, our souls. We confront our demons, we stare the darkest parts of ourselves in the eye, stand toe-to-toe with our inner selves, and learn to accept the dark parts without shame or guilt. There's a seat at the table for the darkness because it's part of us. And we accept it. Our goal is not to create a life without problems, for that would be impossible, but instead to learn how to be fully engaged in our lives. All of our lives. The good, the bad, and the shitshow. We don't justify the actions of our demons, but we do extend them mercy and grace. And something beautiful happens when we extend mercy and grace to ourselves: It becomes easier to extend mercy and grace to others. I don't have this part of soul work nailed yet. There are so many asshats out there who don't get my mercy and grace. But I keep trying.

The alternative to standing toe-to-toe with our inner selves and accepting what we see is to claim victory over our less attractive parts or to ignore them, or worst of all, to feed them. We might indulge in self-hate and guilt. We might hide those parts of ourselves in a closet behind lock and key. Which is tempting because hiding it means avoiding the hard work of accepting it—and make no mistake, the work is difficult and at times can be excruciating. But the only way out is through, and if we don't go through, we remain stuck. There's no shame in being stuck. The first step to getting unstuck is admitting it.

In my early twenties, I was hooked on pornography. I would sometimes forego going out with friends to stay home and watch porn. I would find myself counting down the minutes at work so I could get home to watch porn. I was so ashamed and felt small and pathetic. The shame kept me from confiding in anyone and asking for help. Instead, I told myself it wasn't a problem and that I could control it. Finally one day I decided to talk to a friend about it. I was so nervous beforehand. *Will he shame me? Will he make me feel even smaller? Will he still want to be my friend?* I was so stuck, though, that I had to chance losing his respect and friendship. My friend sat patiently as I tried to get the words out. Once they were out, I nervously waited for him to say something. After what seemed like hours (it was probably two minutes), he said, "I'm glad you told me. What can I do?" My compulsion and shame were no longer locked away in a closet, and my journey to freedom had begun.

I don't believe in a recipe for soul care, but the basic elements are these: knowing, accepting, nurturing, listening, trusting, and then living from soul.

At the age of twenty-two, at the height of my religious indoctrination, I was staring at a fork in the road. I was about to graduate from the University of New Orleans and had two job opportunities. One was associate pastor at my dad's church in Kenner, Louisiana, where I'd lived my entire life, and the second was a pastoral position at a church in Fort Collins, Colorado. As I left my interview in Fort Collins, an older man approached me and asked which job I was going to take.

"I have no idea. I really need to get home and think and pray about this," I replied.

To which he said, "Well, don't stress too much about it. You already know which one you want to do and which one you're going to choose." I was a bit put off by his nonchalant comment, as well as his obvious lack of spirituality and disregard for prayer and inviting God into the decision-making process. And yet, I've never forgotten that conversation—or, more importantly, how I knew in that moment he was right.

How could he know? One word. Soul. He knew that if I were true to myself and listened to my soul, I would have my answer.

This kind of thing has happened for me countless times, as I'm sure it has for you. Faced with a big decision, we wrestle and worry and stress and fret, when more often than not we know deep down what we should do. I'm not advocating carelessness or rash decision-making. I think when it comes to major decisions, we're wise to get alone with our thoughts, and also to discuss the matter with a few trusted companions. However, most of the time our soul has already spoken. We honor our soul by listening.

What could I compare it to? Perhaps to the young man who dreams of a partner to share life with, maybe even a family. He wants that in the deepest part of his being. He desires to be a faithful husband, and he longs to be loved by another with the same desire. He goes on dates, but while many are fun, they don't turn into that. Maybe his ideal relationship isn't possible in these times, he says to a friend. And then just as he begins to lose hope, he meets someone who might be more than fun, more than just a few dates. This person resonates at a deeper place in him, and one day he knows: Yes, this is that. You are them. It is you. It has always been you. He knows it in his bones. He knows it in his soul. And they are married with all their friends and family present for a wedding where the ceremony is short and the party is all night long.

Or perhaps it's like the young woman who doesn't know what gives her life until one day she takes her dad for a physical therapy appointment, and as she watches the therapists interact with her father, something is lit ablaze deep in her being, in her soul. *I was made for this*, she thinks. She puts everything else aside and devotes the next six years of her life to PT school, staying in alignment with the depths of her being, her soul.

This is what it's like when you listen to your soul, when your soul is connected to the Oneness. Soul and Oneness are cut from the same cloth, integral to each other.

In his book, *Let Your Life Speak: Listening for the Voice of Vocation*, Parker Palmer writes, "We will become better [people] not by trying to fill the potholes in our souls but by knowing them so well that we can avoid falling into them." Again, I imagine those early explorers crawling through caves and sometimes finding themselves in very tight predicaments. A passageway that's too small or a hole that's too deep to traverse. They learn from each encounter and avoid making the same mistakes the next day. So is true with our souls. We learn where the pitfalls are, and we learn to avoid them. No need to fear the pitfalls or be ashamed of them. Learn what and where they are. Learn how they trigger and affect you. Know, accept, nurture, listen, trust, and live.

The journey of the soul is no different from cave exploration. Dangerous. Thrilling. Invigorating. Scary. Fascinating. Perilous. And, oh, so worth it. Your life is waiting for you. Your soul is waiting for you.

Life is a beautiful clusterfuck and love is here.
Onward. Forward.*
love.

CHAPTER 5

ALS II

> *"Free, yeah you're on the path and*
> *you tell yourself you need,*
> *You just keep on moving find where you belong,*
> *Life don't last that long."*
> —Anders Osborne; Life Don't Last That Long

As I entered my second year of ALS, I'd completely lost my ability to walk, and my left hand no longer worked, though I could still move my left arm some. I knew I had much more to lose, but I gauged the state of my disease by my ability to eat and breathe, and both were still strong. I felt confident I wouldn't lose my capacity to breathe until year four. My symptoms had basically plateaued for three months, but I could tell things were progressing, and I was somewhat depressed. I was incredibly sad that the disease was moving at a faster rate than I'd anticipated. But despite often feeling sad, I was grateful and excited about love and life. My life was a living, breathing juxtaposition.

By May my right hand also began to lose function. As I'm right-handed, this was a very scary reality. I could no longer grasp utensils or cups, meaning I could no longer feed myself. I could no longer pour my own bourbon, or light my own joints or cigars. I could, however, still hold pizza and tacos and burgers, so I was still winning. And I could still drive my chair, but we had to find a joystick that was easier for me to use.

One day in May, I had to take a poop. Kristy wasn't home, so two of my boys, Micah and Nate, tag teamed to lift me out of my chair, get my pants down, and put me on the toilet. When I finished, I realized I couldn't wipe myself. For the first time. I didn't want to subject the boys to that task, so I asked them to call Margo, our neighbor, who's a nurse. She came over and wiped my butt for me. But then the boys couldn't get me off the toilet, so we had to call our other neighbor, Andy, to assist while the boys pulled my pants back up and put me in my chair. The entire experience was yet another reminder that ALS was intent on destroying me. It was humbling and humiliating and devastating, though also beautiful because my neighbors, my friends, were there for me.

One bright side to my right hand going out was I could no longer bathe myself. Finally, one dream was coming true: Kristy and I would now shower together every day. I'd wanted this our whole marriage. It was going to be amazing! Until, that is, I realized she would keep her clothes on. That was an unexpected plot twist to my dream. Once I moved past disappointment, though, showers became one of our favorite times together. We would put on our playlist and talk and laugh and connect, setting the tone for our day.

Also that spring, my voice weakened and projecting became difficult. We began to meet regularly with my friend and speech-language pathologist, Emily, at Team Gleason. Emily gave me a Britney Spears-style microphone, headset, and amplifier. I hated it because it was uncomfortable and always giving high-pitched feedback. I continued trying to project instead, which proved quite frustrating.

With the kids getting older and developing their own lives, and the rapid nature of my progression, it felt like our family would benefit from a bonding experience, so we decided to take a thirty-day road trip from New Orleans to the western and northwestern US in June and July. This trip turned out to be pure magic for our family.

Our first stop was Amarillo, Texas. From there we made our way to Great Sand Dunes National Park in Colorado, and on to Glenwood Springs, where we soared like eagles as paragliders, a trip highlight.

I've had a fear of heights my entire life, more specifically a fear of falling. At the same time I've always desired to be free as a bird. To my amazement, the entire family wanted to fly, so we set out to be birds.

I was the first to go, and what an experience it was. For starters, it took two guys to get me out of the truck and carry me to the launch zone. Once there, they laid me on the ground, put on my harness, and attached me by the harness to my tandem guide. My four boys got into their harnesses as they watched me being tossed about. Then, someone said, "You ready?" and four guys picked me up and literally threw me over the side of the mountain. Just like that,
I.
Was.
Flying.

I was a raven gliding through the Grand Canyon. One by one, my boys took off, and then all five Jeansonne boys were flying. We felt like kings, invincible, as we soared above the earth's surface, yelling to each other and enjoying our newfound freedom. Once we landed, we watched Kristy and Zoe Moon leap off the mountain. We'll never forget the freedom and joy of being caught between the heavens and the earth.

From there we made our way to what felt like the hottest place on the planet, Moab, Utah, where we visited Arches National Park and Canyonlands National Park. It was in Moab where I had my first of many breakdowns with Kristy about our relationship. One evening we left the kids in the room to sit by the pool together. We hadn't had sex in months, and I felt lonely and frustrated and, most of all, unattractive and undesirable to her. I'd never experienced such insecurities in our eighteen years of marriage. The problem was, she was spent. And we had very different relationships with sex. I needed it; she did not.

I began to cry as I expressed to her how much I missed her body, and how sad and angry I was that I could no longer initiate physical intimacy. My heart broke as I felt the weight of ALS on our relationship. We knew there were more changes to come, changes that would pose potential threats to our relationship. Our future would include interventions like a suprapubic catheter, a feeding tube, and eventually a tracheotomy to facilitate breathing on a ventilator. We could only imagine what these changes would do to our relationship, with Kristy as my primary caregiver. Would she also still be my wife?

Early in my diagnosis, we had a conversation about "tapping out," a term we used to mean letting the disease run its course and stopping the pursuit of further life-extending treatments and therapies. We vowed to be open and honest with each other. Unsure what we were up against, we agreed that if at any point either of us could no longer go on, we were allowed to admit it. I felt so insecure that night, I told Kristy that if she wanted to tap out and let the disease run its course and kill me within the next year or two, I would be okay with that. She was kind and loving as we cried together, reassuring me I wasn't less attractive or less desirable to her, and that she certainly wasn't ready to tap out. Her exact words were, "You better not tap out because these kids will all be grown soon, and there's no one I'd rather spend my time with than you."

We came to no major resolution that night. Our interaction was about seeing and being seen. Like everything else with ALS, we would have to figure out new ways to move forward as situations presented themselves. The talk was therapeutic, and it was also the first time I realized ALS was not only affecting us emotionally; it was changing how we expressed ourselves physically, which would impact our overall relationship. The conversation came at a good time: With the seven of us sharing one hotel room, we couldn't be physically intimate for the next three weeks anyway.

The family surprised me with a second opportunity to go paragliding at our next stop, Salt Lake City, Utah. We then headed to Jackson Hole, Wyoming, where we visited Grand Teton National Park, and continued on to Yellowstone National Park, followed by Glacier

National Park in Montana, and Roosevelt National Park in North Dakota. Our trek back home included stops at Wind Cave National Park, Mount Rushmore, and Badlands National Park, all in South Dakota. Our final stop was the Gateway Arch in St. Louis, Missouri.

My power chair is a beast, so I was able to thoroughly enjoy this trip. On the whole there wasn't much I couldn't do with the family. I would ride the trails as far as I could and then park myself near a river or a waterfall or a rock formation if the rest of the crew wanted to continue hiking or exploring. I kind of liked reclining in a comfortable chair in the middle of nature. I recall a few people walking past me and saying something like, "Now that guy's got the right idea." In total we traveled for 30 days, stayed in 11 hotels, spent 167 hours in the van, and drove 6,523 miles, creating memories along the way that will last us forever.

It's hard to imagine, but ALS could have destroyed our family. Instead, it made us invincible. Kristy and I were determined to shoot for the latter, and it was working, though not without hard work and help. We put one of our kids in counseling immediately upon my diagnosis, and we kept a pulse on each kid as the disease progressed. Eventually all five were receiving therapy. We also continued our custom of playing "mad, sad, glad" at dinnertime. Everyone takes a turn saying something that made them mad that day, something that made them sad, and something that made them glad. As a family, we validate everyone's feelings. The rule in our house has always been, we don't fake it. If you're sad, don't put on a fake smile. If you're mad, don't come around here acting like everything is okay. If you're glad, be happy and don't apologize for it. We carried that philosophy into ALS, with one caveat: I asked the kids to take their lead from me. If I'm not scared, then you don't need to be. If I'm not sad, then you don't need to be. If I'm nervous, then be nervous. At the same time, you can only be where you are, so try to follow my lead but, again, don't fake it.

As the months passed, I felt our family growing tighter. We were gelling and becoming a force to be reckoned with. We had three teenage boys, but we weren't dealing with typical teenage boy rebellion. They were respectful of our decisions as we worked together as a family. I honestly don't know whether we would have shared such a bond at that time in their lives without ALS.

In August 2021, as my voice continued to weaken, Emily at Team Gleason determined it was time to start practicing typing with my eyes on different computers and filing insurance paperwork to get me set up with a communication system. ALS doesn't affect the optic nerves, and Eyegaze® technology allows people with ALS to speak through a computer. I trusted Emily wholeheartedly, as she knew this disease better than I did, and I knew she loved me deeply. Losing my ability to speak was the scariest and most devastating symptom I could imagine. I hadn't enjoyed losing my ability to move and eat, but I ultimately made peace with those losses. Losing my voice was unfathomable, and while I didn't want to face such a reality, I was willing to follow Emily's lead.

As the weeks and months passed, I continued to lose more and more of my right hand. I could still drive my power chair, but I needed someone to place my hand on the joystick. In October we installed an additional joystick on the back of the chair so others could help drive me. It was crushing to feel my autonomy coming to an end. Around this time, I noticed my tongue getting weaker. I had trouble moving food around in my mouth. I also noticed I was having the slightest trouble swallowing. And that's not all.

One of my earliest post-diagnosis symptoms had been sudden urges to pee; when the urge hit, I had very little time to reach a toilet. Peeing my pants became a common occurrence, and at first I was okay with it because, as Billy Madison taught my generation, "It's cool to pee your pants." The dynamics changed as my hands stopped working, though. Now Kristy had to grab the hand-held urinal, undo my pants, and put my penis in the urinal—all before I peed on her.

The game was getting old, and the same month my power chair got its new joystick, I got the first of a few new holes in my body: a suprapubic catheter inserted through my pubic area directly into my bladder. I hadn't even known this was a thing. I'd thought I would have to live with a catheter in my penis for the rest of my life, so I'm sure you can imagine my relief. Yes, I was discouraged to have reached this point in the disease, but the catheter was a game changer and made life easier for our whole family.

The catheter also came with its own share of problems. My bladder apparently wasn't excited about his new live-in guest and began spasming. Imagine having the urge to pee; then, instead of urine coming out, you feel a million razor blades flying down your urethra to the head of your penis. The sensation lasts for several minutes but feels like hours. In terms of penis sensations, the only one you want lasting minutes is an orgasm (which unfortunately only comes in increments of seconds). These spasms were constant, so I finally got my bladder muscles paralyzed with Botox, and it was glorious. I've had Botox injections to my bladder every four months ever since.

The relief was short-lived, though. After the catheter surgery and requisite meds, I became constipated and couldn't poop for five days, a common complication that gets more complicated with ALS. It took them five hours at the ER to confirm what my bowels already knew. They then sent the cutest nurses they could find to administer my enema. Please remember I have ALS at this point and can't move, not even to squeeze someone's hand. Kristy positioned my mouth guard as they inserted the enema so I could clench my teeth against the pain, which was the worst I'd ever experienced. The manipulations took an hour. I couldn't curl into a fetal position for relief. All I could do was lie there and cry. I tried meditating but quickly realized I hadn't reached that level of Jedi Master. I thought for sure I was going to pass out. I begged for drugs, and since it was taking so long, they loaded me up with Valium. I finally shit all over myself.

Needless to say, though I think I've made a good case for it, October 2021 was incredibly difficult.

November brought its own challenges, as my swallowing worsened by the day. I began choking on my pills, and a number of times someone had to pound on my back to force them back up. I could still eat, but eating was exhausting, and I lost weight. Back to the hospital for my second new hole in as many months: a feeding tube inserted into my stomach through a hole in my abdomen. The plan was to feed me breakfast, lunch, and pills through my tube, enabling me to get the calories I needed, and then allow me to eat whatever I wanted for dinner. This was not the worst setup. Everyone knew my eating days were coming to an end, and I milked it. People would call and say, "We want to get dinner for your family tonight. What would you guys like?" For the next few months I ate my favorite meals from my favorite restaurants. Fried shrimp po-boys from Parkway Bakery & Tavern, velvet steak tacos from The Velvet Cactus, Gumbo Ya Ya from Mr. B's Bistro, the Black & Gold Burrito from Juan's Flying Burrito, to name just a few. In addition, my mom and dad, who are the best cooks in the world, came over to cook BBQ shrimp (a New Orleans thing), shrimp Creole, Crawfish Monica, Cajun meatloaf, and a few of my favorite cakes from my mom's repertoire.

In November my computer arrived. I'd decided on the Tobii Dynavox, which runs Windows. I now had in front of my face a computer that would allow me to talk and surf the Internet and watch Ted Lasso and write a book, all with my eyes. The learning curve was steep, so Emily set up solitaire for me to practice on. I began to use my voice throughout the day and the computer to talk in the evenings when my voice was worn out.

Around this time I began needing to use my cough assist and suction more often to clear the junk out of my lungs. First, someone would place a mask over my nose and mouth. Then, once they hit a button on the machine, my lungs would fill with air and the machine would create a powerful suction to pull the mucus out of my lungs and into my mouth, where it could finally be suctioned out of my body. We separated our twin beds so Kristy could more easily reach the machines and help me overnight. It was good for accessibility, but now I was sleeping on an island by myself, and I did not like that at all.

Nights were getting more difficult, and I hated waking Kristy. I vividly recalled the first ten years of our lives together, when she woke every two hours for a crying baby. I just wanted her to be able to sleep. I often got an itch, or perhaps a finger that was uncomfortable. I trained myself to meditate through these minor discomforts so I could save waking her for the big stuff, like coughing. Nothing about this was easy. Training myself to meditate through an itch is one of the more difficult things I've ever done. I lived forty-four years of instant gratification: If I itched, then I scratched. If my leg was uncomfortable, then I moved it, without thinking about it. Now I thought about and felt everything. This was my new life, so I learned to navigate the inconveniences.

When our kids were young, we made a decision to forego gifts for Christmas and instead take a family trip. The idea was stories over stuff. For years, the kids came downstairs on Christmas morning to find their stockings full and a letter from Santa under the tree telling them to pack their bags for a family adventure. On Christmas 2021, our trip was a Caribbean cruise out of Galveston, Texas. Because I required several hands at this time, and we didn't want the kids to have any responsibilities on the trip, our good friend Andrea came with us. The kids had never been on a cruise before. The ship days were amazing as the kids roamed the boat and Kristy, Andrea, and I sat around the pool.

Kristy took the kids on excursion days while Andrea and I stayed back to enjoy the entire ship to ourselves, smoke weed (me, not her), talk, and bask in the sun. On the day of our final port, Kristy and her bestie wanted a girls' day on the beach, so I stayed with the five kiddos. I got a hankering for some real Mexican tacos about an hour into our time together. Anyone who knows me knows that authentic Mexican tacos are my favorite food. I pitched it to the kids: "Hey, let's get off the boat and go find us some tacos." Everyone agreed, so we packed up what we needed and headed to the port, the kids driving my chair for efficiency's sake.

Sometimes when you get off a cruise ship and make your way through the tourist trap, you can find a street with a sidewalk vendor or taco truck, and this is the experience I wanted for the kids. Every time we passed a restaurant I would say, "No, those aren't real, and it's stupid expensive. We want a real taco truck where the tacos are only $2."

We passed restaurant after restaurant but couldn't find the street of my imagination. The kids were getting hangry and tired of my shenanigans, so we circled back and landed at Three Amigos, which happened to be the first restaurant we'd passed forty minutes earlier. The place was expensive, but I told the kids not to worry about it, to get what they wanted. I figured I owed them. We started with the tableside guacamole. I, of course, ordered the tacos even though they weren't the real deal. I sat at the head of the table, and Nate sat to my right; he would take a bite of his food and then give me a bite of mine. We were having the time of our lives, laughing and cutting up, when on my third bite, I literally bit off more than I could chew. As I tried to maneuver the food around in my mouth, it slipped down my throat. At first I thought it was manageable, but then more slid down, and I couldn't breathe.

Micah, our oldest, who was sitting at the opposite end of the table facing me, yelled, "He's choking!" A CPR-certified lifeguard, he leapt into action. All I could think was, *Brian, you have to get this up. You cannot die here in front of your kids.* But I was dying. Nate unbuckled my seat belt and lifted me out of my chair so Micah could get behind me and pound on my back. Jonah ran to call the paramedics. I was sweating profusely, I felt on the verge of blacking out, and I was scared. Jonah took Lucas and Zoe Moon outside when the paramedics arrived. Micah kept pounding on my back, and just as he was about to do the Heimlich maneuver, it came out. All of it. Projected across the table. And I could breathe again.

Micah was overcome with emotion. Jonah, Lucas, and Zoe Moon returned to the table, all visibly shaken. I talked to the paramedics, and Nate sat back down and continued eating. Once everything calmed down, the manager came to check on us and comped our meal. No one was hungry after that, except for Nate, so we left. On our way out Nate said, "Way to go, cheapskate. Only you would go to that extreme to get a free meal."

Again, Steve Gleason's wife, Michel's, words rang true. It's a motherfucker.

I wanted to get close to the ocean to sit and decompress with the kids, so I asked them to drive me there. Micah and Jonah and Nate and Lucas and Zoe Moon—they all thought it was a bad idea. But I convinced them we could do it, so they rolled me toward the water. After about three feet, my power chair got stuck in the sand, and of course it did because power chairs aren't made for sand. Now all four boys had to use every ounce of strength to get me out. I had a mutiny on my hands at this point, the kids deciding it was time they called the shots. We went back to the ship.

The only mandatory activity on that trip was family dinner every evening, during which we went around the table and each told the day's highlight and lowlight. That day had been so traumatic that I made family dinner optional, to give the kids some space. Even so, all five kids showed up at dinner. They wanted to be together. The mood was somber, and for the first time ever I didn't know what to say to my own children.

Micah broke the silence: "How about we go around and give our highlight and lowlight for the day. I know we all have the same lowlight, but maybe we can talk about how we're feeling." Micah began, and then one by one we each bore our feelings. This was one of the most sacred moments I've ever experienced; it felt like we were on holy ground. The vulnerability. The honesty. The tears. The comradery. The empathy. The hugs. The love.

An interaction that completely rocked my world was when one of the boys teared up and said, "I'm so embarrassed because I just froze while you were choking. I was so scared and I didn't know what to do and I hate that about myself." His four siblings got out of their chairs, gathered around him, hugged him, and said, "That's why it's good there are a lot of us. We pick up each other's slack. Next time you might be the one who knows exactly what to do."

And then I had something to say. I went kid by kid and encouraged each of their responses to the incident and validated their individual feelings. We left that table a different family. We were The Jeansonne 7. Some of the kids really had to dive into it with their therapists afterward. We walked through it. Together.

I know those tacos should've been my last meal, but I wasn't ready to let go, so once we were home, I continued to eat one meal a day, resigning myself to puréed food and soups.

For our entire marriage to this point, Kristy and I had enjoyed being on the move, keeping things fresh. Perhaps this is why we had five kids in seven years. We'd owned dogs and rabbits, a hedgehog, and even a pig for a while. Whereas most families move from the city to the suburbs when they have kids, we moved from the burbs to the city. Likewise, when it came to ALS, we kept boredom at bay.

Early one mid-January morning, about twenty months into my diagnosis, as Kristy transferred me from bed to chair, my feeding tube caught awkwardly between us and got pulled out. Kristy tried to reinsert it with no luck, so we packed up and headed to the ER. The doctor I saw there couldn't find a feeding tube, so he inserted a Foley, a much smaller tube, simply to keep the hole open until we could get the correct size. I began to cough as we waited, but as we hadn't brought the cough assist machine, I was unable to cough up what was in my lungs. Thank goodness we were in a hospital, right? Only, every doctor and nurse we asked for a cough assist machine said, "What's that?" *Are you fucking kidding me?* I continued hacking with all my might, and my breathing weakened. Soon the fear set in, and I began to hyperventilate.

Thankfully Kristy had the wherewithal to call the reliable Dr. Kantrow, who knew who to call to get a cough assist machine to the ER stat. By this time I was hooked up to all kinds of machines, and nurses and doctors were flying in and out of the room. It was chaos. My whole body was out of whack. They ordered bloodwork and tried to keep me calm, which kind of worked. My body settled down once a respiratory therapist finally showed up with a cough assist, but my breathing remained labored. Dr. Kantrow arrived just in time to learn my bloodwork results, which revealed that my hemoglobin count was dangerously low for some reason. They began talking about intubating me and giving me a blood transfusion. I asked Dr. Kantrow if this could be it. "We'll do everything we can," he said gently.

Are you for fucking real? Six hours ago I was home completely fine. We only came in because my feeding tube came out.

Dr. Kantrow sensed something was off and ordered new bloodwork. Sure enough, an hour later the new results came back: everything normal. Someone had made a mistake; the first bloodwork results weren't mine. This whole thing was a clusterfuck of magnificent proportions. And not the beautiful kind.

By now it was too late in the evening to have my feeding tube replaced. It had been out for more than twelve hours, which meant an interventional radiologist would need to reinsert it, and specialist doctors had gone home for the day. They sent me to the ICU, where I spent an extremely rough night without my routine medications. At this point in my disease, muscle relaxers were my primary meds.

My body is what's known as "high tone," which in layman's terms means unable to relax, muscles perpetually tense. I was also on meds for depression, Valium for anxiety, and nighttime meds for sleep. But because the Foley temporarily replacing my feeding tube was too small to push meds through, I couldn't take any of them.

Fortunately everything went according to plan in the morning. My body was worn out, though, so they monitored me in the hospital for one more night. The following day as we prepared for discharge, they gave me a Covid test for shits and giggles. Only it was all shit and no giggles, as it came back positive. Everyone pulled on their hazmat suits because now I had the plague, and they transferred me to the Covid unit. It was miserable. I struggled to breathe. Kristy had to give me cough assist every twenty minutes, day and night. The nurses came in the room as infrequently as possible because of the Covid. To add to the drama, none of them was familiar with ALS, so they didn't know how to interact with me. What a terrifying shitshow. If there was a silver lining, it was that we caught the Covid early, which meant I could receive Remdesivir via IV for three days to decrease the risk of serious complications from the viral infection. My cough cleared up quickly, and after five days, I was able to go home.

I spent much of February recovering. My strength for swallowing was pretty much wrecked after my hospital stay.

March of 2022, one month prior to the two-year anniversary of my diagnosis, was hands-down one of the most difficult months for me. It was time to relinquish my autonomy with driving. We removed my joystick. At the same time, I admitted to Kristy I could no longer eat. We picked a day, and at my request, my mom came over to make her chicken and andouille gumbo. I've eaten plenty of gumbos in my life, but none of them compare to my mom's. Though I could only sip a few spoonfuls of the broth, I thoroughly enjoyed my glorious last meal. I can still taste it. This day was also a true joy for my mom. When I was growing up, my mom cooked dinner for our family of four every night, and it always delighted her when my sister and I enjoyed her cooking. There was no question who I wanted to cook my last meal for me. We both won that day.

By April 2022, my anniversary month, I was only squeaking out words. I could say "I love you" with huge breaths between each word. I could kind of say Kristy's name in the middle of the night when I needed to cough: It came out "Kwitty." This was a devastating loss for me. Year two caught me off guard. I think I cried more during that year than I'd cried in all my prior years combined. ALS had stolen everything from me except for the little voice that remained, and my breathing, which felt strong even after Covid.

One thing I continued to do throughout that tough year was sit on my porch. Smoking herb. Conversing with the Oneness. Looking deep inside myself, continuing to know my soul. I pondered what it meant to live a life fully present. I wrestled through grief and suffering. I struggled with comparison and contentment. And I landed on some foundational truths that would carry me through the rest of my life.

Life is a beautiful clusterfuck and love is here.
Onward. Forward.*
love.

CHAPTER 6

ON COMPARISON

> *"Coach, I'm me. Why would I want to be anything else?"*
> —Jamie Tartt*

Not everyone suffers with comparison, I suppose, but I've struggled with it my entire life. It has hindered me from experiencing my true self and, more importantly, from giving the best version of myself to the world. For me, it started young, third grade. Why couldn't I draw like Todd? I loved drawing and tried so hard, but I never could draw as well as Todd, so I quit trying. In middle school, it was: Why can't I be as good a shortstop as Ceravalo? Why can't I make grades as good as Jayme's? In high school: Why can't I hit like Diaz or shoot 3s like Albert? Why can't I make grades like Wolfram? Or get girls like Nuccio? It carried over into adulthood. Why don't my parents have as much money as his parents? It sure would make my life easier. Why can't I philosophize or write as well as Reagan? Or be as enlightened as Nathan? Why can't I let things roll off my back like Crispin? The list goes on and on and on.

The Christian scriptures contain a story wherein Jesus says to his friend Peter, "When I leave Earth, I have some very specific things I want you to do," and then he proceeds to explain what those things are. It's a pretty tall order and a huge privilege, and yet Peter, who suffers from comparison disorder, looks at their friend John who's fishing a ways off, and he asks Jesus, "What about him?" Jesus replies, and I'm paraphrasing here, "Who cares? Am I talking to John? No, I'm talking to you."

Comparison is a thief. When we give in to it, comparison robs us of our sense of purpose and our individuality, and it keeps us from contributing our gifts to society. It robs us of the lives we're capable of living. When we spend our time comparing ourselves to others, contemplating someone else's life instead of directing our time and energy to what we have to offer, we expend energy we'll never get back. We waste precious time. Theodore Roosevelt once said, "Comparison is the thief of joy." Indeed, comparison is another lesson in missing the point.

When I was first diagnosed with ALS, the comparison bug bit me once again, and not in the way you might expect. Rather than comparing myself to healthy people and making my condition more difficult to accept in that way, I began comparing myself to others with ALS. Can you imagine that? I'm diagnosed with a terminal illness, and I actually spend my time searching Instagram and Facebook and Twitter to see how others are doing ALS better than I am. It seemed everyone was doing something extraordinary to advocate for ALS causes.

As I already mentioned, I live three miles from one of the most famous New Orleanians, Steve Gleason, a guy who single-handedly—literally with one hand—lifted the city of New Orleans out of a great depression following Hurricane Katrina by blocking a punt. You see, Steve played for the New Orleans Saints, the city's professional football team. It was September 2006, the first Saints game back in the Superdome and a really big deal. Not only had the city been destroyed a year earlier, but the Superdome itself, where thousands of stranded New Orleanians took refuge during the storm, was also wrecked, both inside and out. The Dome had always been a symbol of hope and strength for a city that lived for its Saints. The Saints are culture, they are soul, they are life in New Orleans. Seeing their home ravaged was a back-breaking blow; conversely, witnessing its coming back to life, renovated and restored, was close to holy.

ON COMPARISON

No disrespect to Steve or any other special teamers (the mostly unknown, unglamorous, underpaid players who take the field during kickoffs and punts), but I'd never heard of Steve Gleason prior to this game, and I wasn't alone. People generally don't know special teamers specifically, just their reputation for being a bit reckless; some, like Steve, have a completely crazy kamikaze approach. So, here's this historic and symbolic game, and the stakes are especially high because the Saints are playing their greatest rival, the Atlanta Falcons, and in the first quarter an unknown special teamer blocks a punt that's recovered for a touchdown, and what follows is perhaps the greatest emotional release ever recorded. Steve is immortalized in New Orleans forever. One play. No one even remembers who recovered the punt for the touchdown. They remember Steve.

Years later when Steve was diagnosed with ALS at the age of thirty-four, the world tuned in. Few people knew much about ALS, but they knew this man had lifted their souls, so they paid attention. And Steve made sure they kept paying attention. This is when he started Team Gleason to help people with ALS access technologies that increase their quality of life. He became an advocate for legislative change, making frequent trips to Capitol Hill to advocate. Steve is the reason I'm able to write this book on a computer with my eyes. I have access to additional tools because of what Steve did with his right hand and then how he used his fame to make a difference.

In 2023, I asked Steve, "I'm curious. If you don't block that punt, do you think your reach and impact on ALS is the same?"

"If I don't block the punt, I would be dead by now," he said.

What Steve meant was that blocking the punt gave him a name and a platform without which he would have been just another statistic, another ALS casualty. Which got me thinking: If Steve doesn't block that punt, I'm probably dead by now too. So, in many ways his right hand saved not only the city's spirit but my life. Can we pause for just a minute and feel the weight of that sentence? Something that happened in 2006, in a professional sports game designed for nothing more than our entertainment, would save my life sixteen years later.

The first time I met Steve in 2023 at the New Orleans Jazz and Heritage Festival (which New Orleanians just call Jazz Fest), I so badly wanted to shake his right hand. But neither of us could move or talk, and our computers don't work outside, so we just stared at each other and tried to smile with whatever facial muscles we had left. As I got to know him better, I learned just how humble and gentle he really is. I don't understand how the universe decides who gets what lot in life—call it chance or destiny or fate or coincidence. (Of course, that's the thing about coincidences, sometimes they just happen.*) All I know is that whatever life dishes out, we're the ones who must decide what to do with it, and Steve decided to use his fame for the good of people like me, and for that I'm forever grateful.

I saw other people with ALS, like Brian Wallach, making similar choices. Brian is a former assistant US attorney who once worked for Barack Obama. He's using his connections in the halls of Congress and the Oval Office to change the face of medical advocacy in the US. In January 2019, Brian and his wife launched I Am ALS, an organization designed to bring people living with the disease and people who love them together to make change. In addition, I Am ALS created a patient-centered movement to fight for research and government funding. Brian's advocacy even led President Biden to sign into law a bill known as the Accelerating Access to Critical Therapies for ALS Act (ACT for ALS), which expanded federal research and gave patients speedier access to treatments still under FDA review.

Steve and Brian might be making a high-profile difference, but when I was first diagnosed and looked around it appeared every average Joe with ALS was doing something, even if just participating in their local ALS walk. *Is this what people with ALS do? Am I supposed to find a gap or a need in the ALS community and fill it?* I didn't block a punt. The closest I got to that was sitting on my sofa in my Drew Brees jersey eating a freshly grilled burger and drinking an ice-cold Abita Amber with friends ten miles from the Superdome. I wasn't even interested in becoming a national advocate—I'd never been one for seeing legislation changed or filling a niche need. Still, I was grateful for every effort I witnessed and began to feel a pressure mounting within me to do something big. What, though? None of it seemed to fit my personality. I felt defeated.

Even in ALS, while actively dying, I was comparing myself to others, and in so doing, I was shaving quality off my life. I knew I couldn't and wouldn't spend the rest of my life in the comparison zone. It was time to decide who I was and what I was for. I was up to the challenge. I'd already been through this a number of times in my life. You know, those times when you look to your gut for guidance?

In second grade, Michael Bouchon and I decided to have a sword fight. The kind when two boys go into the same bathroom stall, unsheathe their swords, and proceed to fight one another with their pee streams. On this day, we both lost control of our swords and ended up peeing all over each other. We agreed not to tell anyone. When we returned to class, Mrs. Ward asked us why our pants were wet, and why we smelled like urine. We looked at each other and didn't say a word. She sent us to the principal's office. I was very familiar with his office, as I spent a good deal of time there and was even paddled by him once. I knew in my gut if Michael and I stuck to our plan, there was no way he could bust us. I was right: We didn't say a word, and we won.

My gut guided me again when I was nineteen and decided to become a Christian and give my life over to following Jesus. And again, when after ten years of pastoring, I asked it whether I'd chosen the right career path. And again for the next six years when I annually asked it the same question. And now at forty-three years old, I was once again asking my gut what to do. This is where all the soul work I'd done became useful. Listening to your gut and listening to your soul are one and the same. The key, as I've mentioned previously, is facing who we are and being willing to truly know ourselves. To understand how we're wired. To familiarize ourselves with our strengths and our weaknesses, and then to learn how to operate in the strengths. The answer I heard from my gut, my soul, this time was that I didn't want to be an advocate. I didn't care about being famous or known in the ALS world. I was, at my core, a pastor.

I took the title of pastor when I was twenty-two. But titles are just that, they don't mean anything substantial, and it wasn't until fourteen years later that I figured out who I was and what I was made for. I figured out I wasn't just a pastor by name. I was a pastor in my bones, in my soul. This is my niche. This is who I am. For clarification, I never considered myself a religious pastor, even though I served as a pastor in a religious context. A religious pastor desires to convert people to their version of God. Look, I know many religious pastors, and they're some of the most gentle and genuine men and women I know. I'm just not them.

My pastoral identity is that of a sojourner, someone who walks through life with others, who traverses the pits and the victories with them. As a sojourner, I have no agenda for anyone else's life beyond journeying with them as they learn to live from their truest self, their soul. As a sojourner, I don't offer answers but presence. I strive to be a sojourner who cares for the well-being of the whole person, who speaks sparsely and listens intently without forming a response while listening. My style as a sojourner is to laugh with people, cry with them, and simply be there with them. Presence.

There's an ancient story in the Hebrew tradition about a man named Job. Job was a good man, respected by others. Out of nowhere, Job's entire life came crashing down on him. He experienced calamity after calamity, including a massive loss of livestock, the sudden death of all ten of his children at one time, and then the loss of his own health. Even Job's wife turned on him. Job, however, had three good friends who came to offer their presence, tears, and love. For seven days they sat in silence with Job, simply being. What a beautiful gift this must have been to Job. True sojourners, friends. Then on the eighth day, his friends opened their mouths and the whole thing went to crap as they tried to explain to Job why these tragedies might have befallen him. One after another they pontificated and philosophized on what Job might have done to bring hardship upon himself.

This is human nature. We desire to offer answers and reasons because we're uncomfortable with uncertainty. Sometimes there are no answers, though, and the best gift we can offer to someone suffering is sacred silence. Upon my diagnosis I'd been practicing sacred silence with others for years. I once heard it said: Let silence do the heavy lifting, the idea being that in silence one is able to connect with their own soul and often to find their truth.

When I lost my ability to speak, sacred silence took on a whole new meaning. I first noticed it with my kids, especially in conversations where I needed to bring correction. While I could speak through my computer, I was limited to speaking only sixteen words per minute. Contrast that to my fourteen-year-old at the time, who could speak 172 words per minute. This is how it went: My kids would come in hot and have to sit there seething while I pecked away with my eyes. I would finally get out a question, they would respond quickly, and I would get back to pecking with my eyes while they sat. A conversation that previously would have lasted twenty minutes and ended with their leaving angry now lasted an hour and offered—no, required—them time to think and feel and cool down. This was the greatest gift I could have ever given my kids, and without ALS I wouldn't have known it. Sacred silence.

I take that dynamic into all my conversations now. Some people are able to tap into the sacred nature of silence, but many aren't. To be quiet with their thoughts is scary; they play on their phones while

I type. But for those who are able to engage, we reach a deeper level together. One where words often aren't needed. The invention of the smartphone, for all its good, has unfortunately robbed us of the art of silence. There was once a time when if we were at lunch with a friend and they went to the restroom, we would sit with our thoughts. There was once a time when we would lie in our beds alone with our thoughts before we fell asleep. We had a built-in sacred silence where our most creative thoughts lived, where we might stumble upon new truths about ourselves.

As I resisted comparing myself to others and tried to figure out what my ALS contribution to the world would be, I realized what I'd long known: That I should play to my strengths and gifts. That I should stay true to my soul and allow it to speak to me, allow it to instruct me on how to best invest in my life, versus allowing my intellect to tell my soul how to live. I needn't strive to be someone I'm not. As Oscar Wilde so brilliantly put it, "Be yourself; everyone else is already taken."

And that's what I did. I realized that my greatest contribution was to offer myself. I began spending my time with people. Sitting. Listening. Creating space for people to come and be. They could talk, or we could just sit. I created space for my friends, for my kids, for my neighbors, and even for strangers. It was a challenge because sometimes I wanted to be doing other things. This book, for instance. The other things, like this book, were good and valid, and I scheduled time for these endeavors, but these other things were not my purpose. I knew what I was for, so I strived, sometimes unsuccessfully, to be present to people, for this was my gift to the world. I know some readers are thinking, "How hard is it to be present when you're already stuck in a chair? You can't leave. How hard is it, really?" Presence isn't a byproduct of physical stillness. Have you ever driven in the car and arrived at your destination only to have no recollection of what route you took or how much time you spent in the car? That's because you weren't present. So, yes, I'm physically confined, but emotionally and mentally I still have a choice.

I'm not the only one who plays the comparison game. I suspect we all desire to keep up with the Joneses to some degree. This desire is a trap; falling into it robs us of our purpose, our lives, our contribution to the world. There is only one you, and you are a gift to this great universe. Learn who you are. Follow your soul. Allow the world to experience you whether you consider your contribution big or small. You are relevant, and the world needs you. Only compare yourself to yourself.

Life is a beautiful clusterfuck and love is here.
Onward. Forward.*
love.

PS: On a Friday afternoon in October 2023, while I was working on the final stages of this book, we received a call asking if we could travel to Washington, DC, to represent Team Gleason and the Eyegaze® technology they provide to people with ALS, at an event called "American Possibilities: A White House Demo Day." In true Jeansonne fashion, we hopped on a plane a few days later, taking two of our boys with us since other caregivers couldn't leave on such short notice. We've never hesitated to take our kids out of school for opportunities, whether it be camping on their birthday or to see a friend in another city, so rubbing elbows with DC bigwigs and touring our nation's capital seemed worth a few days of truancy.

This trip was a step outside my comfort zone and into advocacy territory, though my true motivation for going was the opportunity to give back to Team Gleason, an organization that has given us so much. Once I was there, however, I realized the mission was bigger than just a favor to the team. If the technology that has changed my life can help others, and if I'm able to be the messenger, I will certainly step into that role.

My elevator pitch to people who visited my booth, which I delivered through the computer using Eyegaze®, was as follows:

My greatest fear of ALS was losing my ability to speak. I have five kids, and I was not sure I could handle not being able to communicate with them. If it weren't for the Eyegaze® technology, I don't think I would have chosen to keep living. However, with the technology, I am able to stay in the game of life. I am able to continue communicating with those I love and continue imparting things to my kids. In addition, the technology allowed me to record hundreds of phrases before I lost my voice, and was able to generate a voice that sounds close to my own. Now my kids get the best of me and can still hear my voice. I am forever grateful.

So, advocacy still isn't really my thing, but I'm now willing to step in if called upon.

love.

CHAPTER 7

ON SUFFERING

> *"It's funny to think about the things in your life that can make you cry just knowing that they existed, can then become the same thing that make you cry knowing that they're now gone."*
> —Ted Lasso*

Suffering is agonizing. Suffering devastates. Suffering feels unfair. And not one of us is exempt from it. Some people may get a little luckier in their lives than others, but at some point, we all do suffer. It's a universal bum deal.

From a young age we hear the refrain, "Life isn't fair," and yet somehow we still expect it to be. I like that about us. We're eternal optimists. But then when we suffer, it comes as a painful surprise. *Why me? Why now?* Just, *Why?* All valid questions. As someone who's suffered and asked these questions many times over, I'll offer some answers.

Why me?

If, as we've established, life isn't fair, isn't the better question, *Why* not *me*?

Why now?

Would there ever be a good time?

Why?

Well. Because. Life. Suffering is one of life's fundamental truths; fairness isn't.

But here's another of life's fundamental truths: Suffering can be a wonderful catalyst for transformation and growth. I sometimes wish

I could avoid suffering, and yet I am the person I am today only because of suffering. In my short forty-seven years, I've only experienced true transformation through incredible love and devastating suffering. How's that for a duo?

The greatest source of suffering I experienced prior to ALS was depression. I've been prone to depression for as long as I can remember, dating back to suicidal thoughts in seventh grade. I held the depression at bay for years, but as I mentioned in "On Journey," it was reignited in my early thirties when my dad chose me as his successor to pastor a church of 1,400 people. I'm biologically predisposed to depression, so feeling trapped in work and in life was a trigger. When you have a biological imbalance, it doesn't take much. I desperately didn't want the pastor position, but neither did I want to disappoint my dad or let others in my life down. Life began telling me how to live, instead of me telling life what my soul needed—and by now you know my position on how we should always listen to our soul.

That bout of depression came and went for about four years. Sometimes it hit me for just a day or two, and other times it knocked me out for weeks. Sometimes it was just the blues, but other times it got dark. On those dark days, living felt like trying to breathe underwater without hope of rescue. Hopelessness might be the scariest feeling a person can experience. It's difficult to explain, but this comes close: Imagine yourself in a pitch-black room with no doors or windows, and then the room slowly filling with water. You scream for help, and the water continues to rise. You beg for help, the water continues to rise, and now your head is hitting the ceiling. You realize no one is coming. This is it. At this moment in depression and hopelessness, it doesn't matter how successful you are or how loved you are or how much you have to live for. None of it matters because you're all alone in a pitch-black room, and now the water is seeping into your nostrils, and while you may have people in your life who want to help, none of them can access this room to save you.

This is why people put a gun in their mouth or a rope around their neck or too many pills in their stomach. It's not because they're selfish or weak. It's because they're drowning and alone and hopeless and see no other choice.

This is where I found myself at the age of thirty-seven. I had everything to live for, and yet I was being swallowed alive by the darkness of hopelessness. I didn't get out of bed for days. I had night terrors. One night I woke so paralyzed by fear that I couldn't move. It felt as if the darkness hovering above me was crushing my chest. I was scared almost to death, and I couldn't even call out to Kristy who was no more than a foot away. During this era, I twice went to my closet and picked up my guns just to hold them and think, which scared me enough to ask a friend to take the guns out of my house. It was dark, and I was drowning. Kristy was afraid of what I would do if she left me alone. (Sidenote: At one point, I held a tolerant attitude toward guns. However, as my perspective on violence evolved and my desire for peace grew, my position on firearms underwent a significant transformation. Furthermore, the frequent occurrence of school shootings served as a wake-up call, leading me to contemplate how we, as a society, can protect our most vulnerable. These experiences and contemplations left me with a bad taste for guns.)

I can see now that five things pulled me out of that dark place. My therapist. Medication. My spiritual guide. My Kristy. And my daughter, Zoe Moon.

At around seven o'clock one evening, Kristy came to the bedside and asked if I could find the strength to give our three-year-old daughter a bath. All I had to do was run the bathwater and sit in the bathroom while she played. I rolled myself out of our bed and dragged myself across the room to the bathroom. Zoe Moon was her normal talkative self, while I remained despondent and disengaged.

I sat on the floor and watched her as she played, but I gathered from the concerned look in her eyes that she saw me as only a shell. After about ten minutes she asked, "Papa, what's wrong?"

Tears began to roll down my cheeks. I couldn't speak, only weep. And as I wept, she sat up straight in the bathtub, looked directly at me, and began to sing ...

> *The sun'll come out tomorrow*
> *Bet your bottom dollar that tomorrow*
> *There'll be sun!*
> *Just thinking about tomorrow*
> *Clears away the cobwebs and the sorrow*
> *Till there's none!*
> *When I'm stuck with a day that's gray and lonely*
> *I just stick out my chin and grin and say—*
> *The sun'll come out tomorrow*
> *So you gotta hang on till tomorrow*
> *Come what may*
> *Tomorrow, tomorrow!*
> *I love ya, tomorrow*
> *You're only a day away!*

She was three. That song was not in our playlist. She sang it word for word. That was the night love won. That was the night Zoe Moon saved my life. Say what you will, believe what you want, it doesn't matter to me, but you'll have a hard time convincing me that the universe isn't benevolent and that there isn't something greater than we are—the Oneness—knitting us together in some beautifully interdependent way.

I remember wanting to cancel a meeting with my spiritual guide when I was in the thick of it, and Kristy's not wanting me to. I didn't even have to leave my house because it was a Zoom meeting, and this was before Covid, so Zoom was still a cool thing. I took the call on the back porch wearing my boxers. At one point he asked me, "When this depression lifts one day, how do you think this experience will impact how you relate to people?" In an unfathomable moment of clarity amidst the darkness all around, I responded, "I think I will be more empathetic, and I will have less to say and a greater ability to sit in the suffering of another and simply be with them without feeling the need to fix them." Which is, indeed, what I'm now able to do.

Suffering changes us at a soul level, if we allow it to.

As I look back on that depression more than a decade later, I don't understand how I thought it was so bad. But that's just it. To most outsiders looking in, depression doesn't make sense, and the truth is, depression doesn't make much sense to the depressed person either once they're on the other side of it. I'm no exception. What I know is that when I finally found the light once again, I was a different person. My heart and soul emerged from the deadly, drowning waters, and in a way I felt awakened, as if I'd been reborn. My outlook on life was different. My approach to people had changed. I emerged softer, humbler. I no longer had answers and felt the only gifts I had to offer others were my ears, my life, and my soul. Just myself. Walking with my limp. And for the first time in my life, it felt right. I had nothing to offer but myself and my newfound ability to help others explore the depths and caves of their own souls.

By this time I'd turned away from the position at my dad's church and was pastoring my own. When people called to ask for pastoral advice, I met with them to listen and simply ask questions. I remember one man in particular who came to me for marriage advice. His wife this, his wife that. I asked him questions about himself, and we started digging around in his life and investigating his soul. I could tell he was put off because what he really wanted was for me to fix his wife. But I didn't know how to fix people anymore. I only knew now how to help people think through their own lives and investigate their own souls. The man left our church a few weeks later. Many people would rather try to change others than work on themselves, especially if they haven't done any soul work or prepared themselves for suffering.

That last idea might sound ridiculous: preparing oneself for suffering. But it isn't as out there as it sounds. Remember: We *will* suffer, no question about it. The real question is: *How* will we suffer? And will we waste our suffering, or will we allow our suffering to shape and form us? It's rare to see a person actively searching out ways to learn from suffering while they're in the middle of it. During suffering, we mostly just try to survive. It's possible to train yourself to find beauty in the midst of suffering, but it takes discipline and practice—preparation. To reach the place of recognizing beauty in a period of suffering, we must know our soul. Also important, we must understand that we aren't cursed or victims. Nope. Sometimes we just get unlucky and draw the short straw. The world is full of people who drew short straws. Some of them die victims, and some embrace the hand dealt and play it till their dying breath. It's your choice.

During my depression, I felt like a victim. I wasn't prepared for such devastation, and it nearly destroyed me. Coming out of it, I committed myself to even stronger life practices of silence, solitude, in-depth relationships, meditation, mindfulness, prayer, play, and presence. My hope was never again to be caught off guard. Not that I wouldn't ever suffer again, but I would be more prepared when suffering walked through the door.

And then it happened. Again. Bad news. "Mr. Jeansonne, there is no easy way to say this. This is ALS. I am so sorry."

After a few months, when I was able to breathe again, I found myself bouncing all around the Kübler-Ross stages of grief taught in Psych 101: denial, bargaining, depression, anger, and acceptance. Like an onion, grief has layers. The stages of grief don't cycle in any particular order; nor does grief last for just one cycle. Deep grief

ON SUFFERING

never goes away, it just changes, and over time you learn to navigate life while carrying true sadness and suffering with you in your soul. Forever. It never leaves. It doesn't have to be forever debilitating, but it will never leave. As part of my own grief journey, I one day journaled,

> *I have put a new bench in my soul. I actually created a beautiful garden, with a birdbath, and plenty of bird feeders, plants and flowers and trees. It's quite the oasis for birds and bees, for squirrels and for her. I have come to realize that sadness is here to stay. At first, I thought she would just come for visits, then I began to notice that she was hanging around more often. So, I created a space for her to stay and I wander out to the garden a few times a week and we sit together. There are some things in life that just don't heal. They might sting less over time, but they never go away. So, instead of shaming sadness, I invite her in and even got a really nice bench, as she seems to be a constant companion on this journey.*

I began to emerge from the fog a couple of months post-diagnosis. The doctors gave me two to five years to live, so I began contemplating how I would live them. I sat on my front porch for countless hours, thinking. If I'd learned anything from my bouts of depression, it was that all is never lost, and hopelessness doesn't last forever. More importantly, it taught me that the pathway to depth and maturity and wisdom and contentment travels downward, into the deep recesses of the soul.

No one—and there's no exception to this—no one reaches the top of the mountain without first experiencing the utter depths of the canyons. There exist only two paths to change and transformation, and they're the paths of great love and great suffering. Those with eyes to see and ears to hear know this truth in their bones, in their soul. They wear it in their bodies. Pain and suffering are the most brutal motherfuckers, and if you hold on, they will also be the most formative. Don't fool yourself into thinking you can escape unscathed: You won't endure great suffering and come out the same on the other end. It's your choice whether the suffering forms you for the better or for the worse.

So, how has the suffering of ALS formed me? I suppose this question would be best answered by those who know me, but they aren't here in my living room this afternoon as I write, so I'll give you my own take on me.

Since my major depression, and now ALS, I feel lighter. I no longer feel I have anything to prove, and I'm able to approach life more openhandedly. I don't feel a need to be right. I'm only willing to sell out my soul for one thing, and one thing only: love. I don't have as much to say. I listen better, and I don't pretend to understand. I see life as a mystery and nonlinear. "I'm sorry" comes more easily, as does "I forgive you." Certainty is not a thing, and the world is full of magic. More than anything, suffering has given me new eyes to see people. And to love them.

People often compare their suffering to mine; they tell me about their suffering and then say, "Then I think about you, and I'm like, my problems aren't anywhere near what you're going through." That bums me out. Why would someone feel the need to compare, and in so doing dismiss their suffering? (See "On Comparison.") Suffering is suffering. It's where you are. And yes, if it were a competition, I would win nine out of ten times, as even among healthcare providers, ALS has the reputation of being the cruelest of all diseases. But it's not a competition. Don't dismiss your suffering. Unless you're suffering because first class was full, so you had to fly economy. I know six people who have lost loved ones since my diagnosis. Five lost children (aged nine, sixteen, seventeen, thirty-one, and a newborn at birth). Another lost her husband, a father of four children under thirteen years old. I make no claims to know their pain. How could I? And they don't pretend to know mine. When we get a chance to sit together, we hold hands and look into one another's eyes, and we're quiet. Because we speak the same language of brokenheartedness and loss. And we know there's no fix to the pain. We look to each other for solidarity, for companionship, for safe space, and for love. We don't need words because, honestly, there are no words that ease the hurt. We allow the presence of the other to validate our brokenness, and we feel seen.

No one asks for it. Suffering is an uninvited guest. It will humble you and make you reliant on others. But it can also shape and form you for the better. Don't waste your sorrows. Give yourself plenty of grace, and sit with sadness whenever she visits. Be kind to her. Don't shame her. Honor her, offer her a cup of coffee.

Life is a beautiful clusterfuck and love is here.
Onward. Forward.*
love.

CHAPTER 8

ON TRAINING

> *"Taking on a challenge is a lot like riding a horse, isn't it? If you're comfortable while you're doing it, you're probably doing it wrong."*
> —Ted Lasso*

In 2009, at the age of thirty-two, I developed a passion for running. Up until that time, I hadn't understood running or the people who engaged in it. But I needed a reprieve from my anxiety and the chaos of my mind, so I took up running. I trained hard and ran my first race ever in February 2011, the New Orleans Rock 'n' Roll Half Marathon, finishing in 1:49. I ran several halves that year, eventually setting a personal record in the hills of Nashville with a time of 1:41.

I felt so strong at the end of the half marathons, like I could easily run 13.1 more miles, so in 2012 I signed up for my first full marathon. I thought I would just keep the same training program I'd been using for the halves; on race day I'd simply tag on the extra miles. I told a friend who'd already run a marathon my plan. He encouraged me to do at least a few longer runs, maybe one sixteen-miler and one eighteen. I could see the wisdom of his advice. On my first sixteen-miler, I was cruising right along. Miles thirteen and fourteen were a breeze. Then at mile fifteen, my body started to revolt. My legs turned into soggy spaghetti noodles, and my breathing became labored. At that moment I realized I couldn't half-ass the front end and expect a positive outcome. So, I set my sights on a positive outcome and committed to training. To run a 26.2-mile race, I would first need to run hundreds of training miles.

And that's exactly what I did. For four straight months, I ran and ran and ran some more. I was on pace to run a sub-four-hour marathon. My goal was 3:45, and I was confident I could do it. Then one morning, on one of my short five-milers, I felt a twinge in my knee followed by an excruciating pain, as if someone were stabbing the side of my knee with a knife. I couldn't run more than 3.3 miles before the stabbing feeling would begin. So, one month before the race, I had to lay off my knee and stop training.

I never once considered bowing out of the marathon. As race day approached, I had no idea what to expect. I hadn't run for a month. I was still in excellent cardio shape, as I'd continued high intensity interval workouts for that final month, but that's not running. The morning of the race, I woke up excited and ready. I arrived at the starting line completely jazzed, my playlist set to crush the course. The horn sounded, and we were off. It felt easy. Effortless. I was doing it. My knee felt fine when I hit the 3.3-mile mark. Yes! And then, at 3.5 miles, the knife pierced my skin. I could feel it in my bone. Little sucker tricked me. I faced my first big decision of the race: Quit now or run? I queued up Eminem's "Lose Yourself," and I ran. And I cried and cursed and hurt. But I ran anyway. I'd worked too hard to quit. Around the 5.5-mile mark the pain began to subside, and by mile six it was gone altogether.

Game on.

I had some time to make up, but I could do it. When I got to the spot where full marathoners veer to the left and half-marathoners split in another direction, it was again decision time. I felt great. Veer left. I ran, the cool February New Orleans air gliding over my freshly shaven head. For the next four miles I was invincible—at least until mile seventeen. That's where the wheels fell off, as well as the muffler, the transmission, and some other parts I didn't recognize. I was dehydrated and cramping in both quads, hamstrings, and calves. The cramps played musical muscles for that mile. Finally, at mile eighteen, I guzzled sixteen ounces of salty Gatorade and ate a few more salt packets at a medical tent, but my hopes for a sub-four were dead. All my training. Hundreds of miles. Countless hours. Dead at mile seventeen. Oof. Turns out that last month of training is critical. I cried and I cursed and I faced another decision: Quit now or finish?*

As part of my training for the marathon, I'd built in breaking points, or what my military buddy calls "mindfucks." On a sixteen-mile run, for example, I would intentionally route myself to run past my house at mile thirteen or so, to give myself the option of calling it quits. The point being, I'd even trained for this moment of truth in the marathon. Sure, my dream of finishing in 3:45 was dead, but I still needed to finish the race, for me. And those built-in mindfucks turned out to be invaluable. I knew how to resist their temptation and keep going.

I think it was around mile twenty-one, while I was on my way up a bridge, that a cute little old lady, easily in her late seventies, passed me like I was standing still. The worst mindfuck yet. I struggled through the next several miles, but somehow the final stretch was like running on clouds. I crossed that finish line four hours and forty-nine minutes after I'd started, weeping. I hugged Kristy and wept some more.

Training. It's hard work. It's time-consuming. It's not always fun. It costs you: time, energy, effort, sweat, tears. Training for a marathon means waking up at 4:00 a.m. to run in rain, sleet, freezing temperatures, and sometimes sunshine. It means sore muscles and ice baths. You do, though, reap rewards when you put in the work. The rewards for me in marathon running were crossing the finish line and, more importantly, learning how to work through pain and heartache and disappointment and keep going.

Around the time I started running and training my body, I also began training my inner life. The exact order of events is a bit fuzzy, but in my early thirties I was exposed to the book *Emotionally Healthy Spirituality: It's Impossible to Be Spiritually Mature, While Remaining Emotionally Immature* by Peter Scazzero, which addresses getting in touch with emotions instead of avoiding them. It introduced me to a more holistic approach to paying attention to and taking care of my inner life—mind, soul, emotions, all of it. I'd already had a lifetime of religious teachings to guide me, but emotions weren't prioritized or even addressed in my religious upbringing. I can even say that, in my experience, most religious people seem to view emotions in a negative light. Perhaps they see emotions as hindrances to accessing God. In any case, Scazzero's book sent me on a journey of learning more about myself. Some of us at our church at the time started a class on the book to dig in more deeply. We were called "humanist" by people in other churches, and even by some in our church, in a derogatory way. See, people become scared of what they don't understand, and our willingness to think outside religious doctrine was threatening.

Me, though, I couldn't get enough. I kept going after the class at church ended. I didn't know anyone personally who practiced the type of spirituality I was being drawn to—one of quiet reflection, prayer, contemplation, stillness, calm—so I read more books and began integrating their practices into my life. Meditation, mindfulness, centering, sitting in silence, contemplation, solitude, rest, and therapy. I eventually found an organization called Sustainable Faith with cohorts all around the country in which people gathered for two years to study ancient spiritual practices. The two years I studied with Sustainable Faith were difficult, scary (remember how what we don't understand can be scary), time-consuming, fun, boring, and exciting, and they opened me up to a beautiful new way of experiencing life and spirituality.

Which brings me back to training. If you really want to know who you are, spend some time by yourself in the quiet for hours and hours. We live in a society that values being busy. Ask someone what they've been up to, and you almost always hear something like, "Oh, you know, just been busy." As if it's a badge of honor. I suppose if they were to answer, "Not much. I work as little as possible and spend the rest of my time with my friends, family, and neighbors," we'd judge them for being lazy or unmotivated. We might envy them, but we probably wouldn't admit it.

One of the greatest gifts of ALS is that I'm not busy.

"Brian, what have you been up to?"

"Oh, you know. Mostly just sitting around, only doing things I want to do." And nobody gives me shit about it.

In many ways, getting to know one's inner self is like training for a marathon. However, inner life training is more sustainable; the effects last longer and pay huge dividends when you least expect it.

Hence, we train. We practice. Practice? We're talking about practice?* Yes. Practice and training. We often choose not to because practice and training require quieting our minds, and our heads can be scary places. So, instead of getting quiet, we placate our heads with food or music or podcasts or wine or whiskey or weed or painkillers or masturbation or spending money or sex or anything that takes us away from our inner lives. An enormously large percentage of people throw themselves into work and find their identity there. Anything not to be alone with ourselves.

We were made for more than this, though. We were made for more than living out our lives in empty shells. And to live the lives we were intended to live, we must train.

People frequently ask me how I handle having ALS so well. "I just don't think I would be able to do it," they say.

To which I ask, "What practices do you engage in to take care of your soul?" And, "How often do you practice silence and solitude?"

If they answer nothing and never, then I agree they probably wouldn't be able to handle ALS like I do. The good news is it's never too late to start. Plus, if you get ALS tomorrow, you'll have two to five years to get the hang of it. ALS has been the biggest mindfuck of my life, no doubt. And yet, when I was diagnosed at the age of forty-three, I was ready. In many ways I was made for this. I'd been training.

So, how does one start? How does one recognize their own soul? And how does one follow it?

As I've mentioned previously in this book, it feels presumptuous to offer a prescription for anyone else's inward journey. This isn't a how-to book. It's true, though, that I've come a long way from my God-fearing, evangelical Baptist upbringing, and most days I do feel like I'm journeying okay with ALS. It would be insincere to pretend I have no advice to offer, so here comes a bit of direction.

For beginners in training, my first recommendation is to avoid adding one more obligation to an already busy life. Our plates are full. We work full-time while squeezing in workouts and being there for our kids' gymnastics tournaments. We spend countless hours in carpool lines and work three jobs while caring for elderly parents and making space for passion projects and hobbies. All of these things matter. Don't let any of them go, even for soul care. Instead, start by integrating the small practice of just being into what you already do. When you're in carpool line, turn off the radio, put your phone away, and just sit. When you're on the treadmill, turn off the music, and just run. When you're alone, resist turning on the TV or picking up a book, and just be there. When you relax on your porch in the evenings with a cigar and a bourbon, or when you take a hot bath, just do those things. No podcast. No texting. No mindless scrolling. Soak with your thoughts. Be with yourself.

From here, I suspect you'll begin to think about integrating other new practices into your life. Practices like meditation, prayer, contemplation, silence, solitude, not speaking, and more. The urge will arise organically, but you must start small to get there. Otherwise, soul care becomes a Get Your Inner Life Right in Just 30 Days kind of stunt. When taking care of your inner life does become more of an intentional practice, think about building your life around rhythms of silence and solitude. The rhythm of journaling twenty minutes each day as you process your thoughts. The rhythm of regular thirty-minute walks without headphones. The rhythm of guided meditations, especially ones that teach mindfulness and consciousness. If prayer is already one of your daily rhythms, try cutting out the speaking element of prayer and shift to prayers of listening.

I always ran better with music when training for races, but I did build in the practice of taking one five-miler a week without music, simply to reflect on my life and listen. As my understanding of Oneness evolved, I came to believe that Oneness doesn't intervene in lives by answering specific prayers, like *God, please heal me*. Prayer became even easier because I no longer had anything to ask; I simply needed to be and listen.

I have to be honest, though, and admit that training never ends. There are many days now when I would rather watch "Ted Lasso" or listen to music than take the time to be by myself or to meditate. But I know the benefits, so I keep training.

Learning about and listening to your inner life, your soul, is the most important work you can do. It takes time, energy, perseverance, commitment, and patience. Lots of patience. People often don't understand or practice the art of a slow life because they don't see the benefits quickly enough. Humans want checklists and instant results. That's why we go for quick fixes for losing weight or gaining muscle; why we want to master the guitar in a month or basket weaving in just five easy steps. But in soul training there are no quick fixes. No shortcuts.

It can be a scary venture, to be alone with our thoughts. To come face-to-face with ourselves. Our deepest parts. Our shadow selves.

Most of us don't live as our true selves; instead we live in a way we believe others will approve of and accept. We live as our imposter or our poser. Sometimes it's called the false self or the glittering image. I prefer Carl Jung's term, shadow self.

As a friend once told me,

> *When I look at you, I see what you want me to see,*
> *When you look at me, you see what I want you to see.*

We develop this shadow self at a young age as a way to survive in a cruel world. We learn what's acceptable and what's unacceptable, whether from our parents or our teachers or our peers. We figure out how to fit in by suppressing our true selves. We operate instead from our insecurities, our wounds, our hurts, and our failures. In some ways, this is what I was doing in my role as associate pastor at my dad's church. I was changing on the inside and feeling a tension growing, but I didn't want to hurt or disappoint others. Eventually the tension became too tight, I could hardly breathe, and I realized I needed to be true to myself and branch out.

The shadow self isn't bad or good. It's just part of us—it's everything about us that lurks in our subconscious. As we train and get to know ourselves better, the shadow emerges, and that allows us to work on ourselves at a deeper level. It may be difficult not to view your shadow self as inherently bad, but consider this: In the Taoist tradition, distinctions between good and bad are perceptual, not real. Thoughts of lust and anger are not bad, and feelings of kindness and gratitude are not good. Yin and yang comprise an indivisible whole. When we disregard dichotomous moral judgments, we free ourselves from the shackles of shame and guilt, as well as the euphoria of feeling pride in ourselves; we're then free to explore the nature of our thoughts and to determine for ourselves who we want to be.

Sometimes our shadow self protects us; other times it hinders us from being known. I'm sure you've noticed your shadow self showing up—that time you were only pretending to understand what someone was talking about, or that time you received a promotion and got in way over your head, or that time you apologized to help someone else save face even though you weren't in the wrong.

One recess when I was in fourth grade, a soccer ball hit my thumb and jammed it. As if a hand ball giving the other team a free kick wasn't bad enough, I started crying. And then my part-time friend/part-time bully made fun of me for crying. That was the day I learned crying is a sign of weakness, and that all people who cry are weak. For the next two decades, my shadow self protected me from being perceived as weak by keeping me from crying. My shadow self also inflicted emotional pain on others by interpreting anybody else's tears as a sign of weakness. I didn't figure this out until my early thirties when a woman who I supervised in my pastoring role began to cry during one of our meetings. "There's no reason to cry over this," I told her. She looked me right in the eye and asked, "Why does my crying make you so uncomfortable?" I didn't know why, and her question sent me down the path of self-exploration.

We aren't made to live dualistic lives. We're made to live in wholeness and harmony with ourselves. We're made to live from our souls, our essence, our true selves. The only way to do this is to recognize and befriend our shadow self. As Jung writes in *The Archetypes and the Collective Unconscious*, "The meeting with oneself is, at first, the meeting with one's own shadow. The shadow is a tight passage, a narrow door, whose painful constriction no one is spared who goes down to the deep well. But one must learn to know oneself in order to know who one is."

Knowing, accepting, and loving ourselves is of utmost importance, for without this we can never really truly love another. You're probably familiar with the Golden Rule: Treat others the way you want to be treated. Philosophers, poets, artists, and teachers have taught the lesson in many ways. The ancient Greek philosopher Aristotle believed loving yourself is integral to loving others. In his work, *Nicomachean Ethics*, Aristotle writes, "The defining features of friendship that are found in friendships to one's neighbors would seem to be derived from features of friendship toward oneself. For a friend is taken to be someone who wishes and does goods or apparent goods to his friend for the friend's own sake."

Another great philosopher and teacher, Jesus, who was likely familiar with Aristotle's teachings, simplified it even more by saying, "Love your neighbor as yourself."

How can we treat others the way we think we should be treated or love others as ourselves if we don't know and love ourselves, every single thing about ourselves, even the stuff we don't like about ourselves? Just as we must accept everything about our soul, we mustn't shame our shadow self. We must instead accept our shadow self with loving kindness. We can't love other people the way they deserve to be loved if we don't love and accept ourselves because we end up despising in others what we hate in ourselves. We must know how we deserve to be treated before we treat others the way we deserve to be treated. The only way we can get to where we want to be is by getting to know ourselves, our souls. So, we train.

I've found this to be so true in my own life. When I was addicted to pornography, for instance, my shame made me insanely judgmental of other people with the same addiction. At times when I've most despised the part of me that has an incessant need to be right all the time, I've also been intolerant of other people who need to be right. When I've craved attention and needed to feel important, I haven't been able to stand other people who desire the limelight. What I've hated most about myself throughout my life, I've also despised in others. And what Aristotle and Jesus and so many other wise people have written and said rings true. It took recognizing these qualities in myself, and accepting them and

ON TRAINING

extending love to my whole self, for me to be able to extend grace to others and love them more fully.

I trained for five months to run 26.2 miles. It was grueling, invigorating, full of highs and lows, transforming to my physical body and my mind. The journey inward is different. It takes a lifetime of training whenever you start. Why not begin now? It's hard work, but as my dad always says, "If it were easy, everyone would be doing it." It's the kind of work that will slowly transform your life as you put one foot in front of the other day after day, month after month, year after year. Build in your mindfucks. Put in the time. Wave at the old ladies passing you on the left. Our lives depend on it, and our souls are waiting for us.

Life is a beautiful clusterfuck and love is here.
Onward. Forward.*
love.

CHAPTER 9

ON PRESENCE

*"Living in the moment is a gift.
That's why they call it the present."*
—Ted Lasso*

Space and place. That's where we live every moment of our lives. Our physical body can only occupy one space in one place at any given time. In this precise moment as you read or listen to this book, your physical presence is occupying a space in a place. Are you here for it? Perhaps a better question: How often are you not here for it? Imagine you're at the movies with a friend. Your physical body is inarguably sitting in the theater seat, and your eyes are looking at the movie screen, but unless the movie is at a point of high tension or drama, chances are your thoughts are in a million other spaces and places. While the movies ought to be a reprieve from the chaos of life, we stuff a backpack with all our worry and anxiety when we head to the theater. We may as well save the $12 and sit home with the bottle of Blantons we just bought. One space in one place is what you get—it's your decision how much of you shows up for it.

Here's a bit of truth: Those who commit to practicing being right here right now, the people who learn to be in the present, live light and free and dance whimsically with life.

Don't think for a minute, though, that learning to live in the present comes easily. No. This is more hard work, more training. They won't teach you presence in staff meetings or in class at university. You might find a workshop on living in the present, but your certificate of completion will be meaningless. You're going to have to take this on personally. You'll need to dabble in some monk or yogi or Jesus or Jedi shit. This is a journey into the sacred. We're talking about holy ground kind of stuff. There's no magic presence pill, no Thirty Days to Become a More Present You program. Presence takes years and years of practice. A lifetime of commitment and devotion. The ability to be present is what separates those who go through the motions of life from those who truly experience life. It's what separates the mystics from the rest of us.

It may sound like an unattainable goal, to be a mystic, but plenty of mystics walk among us. They're the people who find love and life, beauty and mystery, everywhere they go. Mystics live with a quiet confidence, and they not only feel peace, but they are themselves a peaceful presence. The mystic recognizes the beauty and love in life during the good times and the tragic times. The mystic is content in all circumstances—not because they were born content, but because they work at contentment. The mystic is inquisitive and curious. The mystic doesn't need answers or proof, for the mystic is connected to the Oneness and understands that answers and explanations are nothing more than humans trying to make the infinite finite—which stands in direct contrast with flowing in the beauty and mystery of love and life. The mystic doesn't concern themselves with what's right or wrong, but instead with what's love. The mystic is connected to self, others, and the Oneness, fully aware that all is interdependent.

The life of a mystic takes practice and commitment and conviction, and as Friedrich Nietzsche once said, it demands a long obedience in the same direction. When a person walks this path, they understand that to be truly and fully present is the point, as now is the only moment life can be experienced. And experiencing life is why we're here. The mystic's feet are firmly planted in the soil of this life with all its ups and downs. Life doesn't give the mystic special treatment or more triumphant moments; nor does it protect the mystic from tragedy. The mystic lives in the world just as everyone else does, though the mystic has new eyes for seeing the world and existence for what it is. The mystic lives in the tension of light and darkness, evil and love, yin and yang, with a soul deep enough to sit empathetically with the most horrific pain and wide enough to hold the joy of a billion brides. The mystic does not see in black and white, but in full color. The mystic's life is spacious. The mystic knows love and journeys deeper into it as each day passes.

I remember so clearly the moment I clumsily stumbled upon the truth of living in the present. At the beginning of a session with my counselor, he led me through a guided meditation. He prompted me to check in with my physical presence and at some point asked me, "How do your elbows feel?"

I had no idea how my elbows felt. A thirtysomething man and I'd never once thought about how my elbows felt. Except that one time during a varsity baseball game my junior year when I caught a wayward fastball on my left elbow while at the plate. Of course, my having never considered my elbows was the point of his question: He was asking me to be present, in my body, in a particular place, while occupying a space at a precise moment in time.

The mystics and the others who have learned that life can only be experienced now also know that worry is a thief that aims to overwhelm and steal your passion and zeal for life. What is worry? Is it not projecting a potential negative outcome on a future scenario that we have little, if any, control over? Worry comes when we leave the present. Worry arises when we allow an undetermined future to take up space in our minds. Here's a bit of truth: Plenty of things will go wrong in the future; no need to leave the present and project anything else.

The squirrel is one of my favorite animals. I love watching them scurry around the great oaks that shade New Orleans. One thing I've noticed about squirrels is they never seem worried. They don't seem to concern themselves with whether there will be enough acorns for dinner; nor do they seem to wish they were instead a magnificent oak. No, they seem content with being squirrels. Doing squirrel things. Trusting that at dinnertime they'll figure it out and the universe will show up and provide once again.

I sometimes used to sit for hours at my neighborhood coffee shop on Esplanade Avenue, watching the squirrels play. Jumping from tree to tree, dancing effortlessly across power lines, chasing each other, and perching on a limb to watch the humans coming and going. I often wondered, *Do these squirrels look down on us from their perch on those great oak limbs and envy our human experience of life?*

The squirrel probably doesn't possess the ability to think such thoughts. But as a squirrel-watching (and people-curious) human, I would bet the house on it that if the squirrel had reflective thoughts, it would say, "No, I don't want to be human. Unless I can be that older, dark-haired dude with the big, black-framed glasses and big gut. He's always laughing and carrying on and doesn't seem bothered by much. I'd switch places with him. Or the one that sits inside—we can see them through the window, always sipping their coffee as they create comic book characters. Yeah, there's a depth to that one. Or the guy in the white Chucks who always asks for a mug instead of a paper cup. You know, the one who smells his coffee before savoring the next sip; he just sits there enjoying his coffee as he watches us. As for everyone else, it's too much hustle and bustle. These people, scurrying around, in and out, move, move, move to the next meeting, using their coffee as a pick-me-up to help them get through their morning. I'm glad it works for them, but I'd rather keep my squirrel life."

You see, the only moment that matters to the squirrel is the moment it's currently living. Humans, though, have the unfortunate ability to be in a hundred places at one time. Of course, this ability can sometimes be a useful curse, but usually it's a thief intent on stealing the gift of the present from us.

We human beings do, however, have the capacity to train ourselves to live and be present to the moment. It just takes work.

ON PRESENCE

In my early twenties, I realized I needed time alone to take care of myself. During this period, I developed a practice of journaling, as well as a practice of spending time by myself in silence and stillness. In those early years, I didn't have a target, and I didn't know there was anything unique about these practices. I figured everyone must do it, if for no other reason than to maintain sanity.

I soon noticed while journaling and being quiet that my insides and my outsides weren't in sync. If anything, my outsides—my circumstances—were messing up my insides. I didn't think it should be so. I wanted a life where my insides were in charge, my inner life determining how my outer life operated. This is when I decided to pay even more attention to my insides. My soul. (If you're reminded of "On Soul" and "On Training" here, that's by design. It's all connected.)

It didn't take me long to grab a sledgehammer, as I began to crave and then pursue an integration of my whole being. I longed to be able to live lightly and freely in all areas of my life, even when life got shitty. I began taking my inner life more seriously by learning how to meditate more deeply, learning how to pray without attachment to outcome, learning mindfulness, and learning how to reflect upon and examine my life. I learned how to center myself in space and place, as well as how to surrender to life. Above all else, I learned how to sit alone in silence with just me and my thoughts. Quiet. Silent. Sacred.

My job as a pastor afforded me time for this type of internal work. My primary job description was to care for those in my congregation, to walk through life with them, and to show and teach them how to take care of their inner life. Simply put, I saw my job as teaching people to find, develop, and nurture their soul to the degree that they would no longer "need" church. The truth is, you can't lead others into territory where you haven't been. So, I devoted hours a week for years to nurturing and caring for and getting to know my soul, and learning how to listen to it.

Early on I realized that the disparate parts of my inner life—emotions, ego, values, etc.—existed inside of me in silos, never associating with each other. Each part steered clear of the others. Compartmentalizing all my parts kept me safe because they couldn't challenge each other and cause tension, and it allowed me to live an imposter's life because an unintegrated life is an imposter's life. But an unintegrated life, an imposter's life, takes energy. I grew tired of my internal structure, so I renovated. These silos in my mind's eye were each made of malleable metals, which made them easy to tear down. I then repurposed the raw materials to build instead a huge, round table and enough chairs to accommodate all my parts. At this table everyone (all my parts) gets a seat and a voice. There's no head of the table. All of us (me and my parts) eating and drinking together became a regular practice. I would get quiet, and we would gather around the table and share gut-level feelings, thoughts, struggles, and questions.

Upon entering the dining hall, my parts and I would check in, get our name tag and our cane, look for our place card, and take our seat at the table. We didn't always sit in the same seat. Parts that needed some deeper connection with and understanding of each other would sit close so they could hash things out. There was always small talk as we settled in. It was awkward in the beginning, as none of us had ever met before.

There were seats for Sadness, Anger, and Envy. There were seats for Love, Mercy, and Grace. Addiction got a seat, as did Judgment. The part of me that liked watching Pornography and the part that felt Shame over it both got a seat. As you might guess, those two usually sat next to each other because we were always trying to iron stuff out. There were seats for Guilt, Embarrassment, Joy, Fear, Happiness, and Resentment. There was also a seat for Insecurities, as well as Pride. There were more, but those are some of the heavy hitters.

We would gather for hours, enjoying our meals and getting drunk on wine and whisky. There were a few beer drinkers, as well as two who drank those fruit-flavored hard seltzers, but even they felt comfortable because this was a no-judgment group—which was challenging for Judgment, but he honored our agreement. The group was founded on honesty, trust, loyalty, humility, and love. We all got canes at check-in because here we all walk with a limp. Some parts did all they could to hide their limp, any sign of weakness. Everyone enjoyed watching Pride walk with a cane in those early years; it was so difficult for him. Arrogance had the same hang-up, but eventually life kicked the shit out of both of them. It was bad. Pride was in the hospital for weeks, but you know what? He got so comfortable with the cane that he decided to use it all the time. Pride finally realized the cane wasn't a sign of weakness at all but rather of strength and survival, maturation, and wisdom earned.

After dinner, some of us would enjoy a cigar. Others smoked cloves, and of course Stress and Carefree always shared a few bowls. We would go around the table and rate our current pulse on a scale of one to ten, and then unpack the rating for the group. Reports would be short for some of us, while others who felt defeated or worn out would get the floor for however long they needed. The beauty these gatherings elicited is impossible to put words to. When Sadness bore all her distress and heartbreak, how could Envy and Judgment not absorb it and grow in compassion and love? When Sadness finished speaking, we didn't jump in with comments. We validated Sadness's feelings by holding her story in our souls. *We see you, Sadness, and we love you, and we are you as you are us.*

After some time, we broke our sacred silence with a toast to Sadness, and then we moved on to witness a story from another part of the whole.

Now Pornography had something to say. On this night they were sad. They liked watching pornography and masturbating because it helped relieve stress, but the vibe was sad because life was crushing their wife. She was overwhelmed and couldn't turn the sex switch on. She was tapped out at night, all the parts saw it and weighed in on it—they remained open, and no conversation or thought was off-limits. To ask her for sex at night would put her in the difficult and precarious position of finding some magic sexiness potion or, worse, saying no and then wearing the guilt of not doing enough. This was a difficult season in their lives, and he missed being with her. He longed for her. She said she was okay with masturbation, so he engaged pornography and masturbated. Depending on how you were raised, you're either in the "yeah, cool" camp or the "this is disgusting behavior" camp. Both camps masturbate, but one camp can't talk about it and condemns it. Actually, that's how most of the other parts felt about Pornography before these no-judgment discussions. (To alleviate confusion, this was in my pre-ALS days. After ALS, the penis is still fully functional but your hands are not, so I'm sure you can imagine the conundrum.)

Once Pornography finished speaking, we held their story in our soul in sacred silence. We could clearly see that Shame had been moved by the story. As had Judgment, Guilt, and Love, who integrated Pornography's narrative into themselves because they are them. At our table, we're all integrally connected to one another and to the Oneness. Then we toasted Pornography and gave the floor to another part of the whole.

We never offered advice to the other parts, and we didn't try to fix each other. We gathered to acknowledge one another and offer a space for honesty and vulnerability, without Fear of Judgment taking over. Each part became known by all the others. We developed a rich and deep and compassionate love for one another. As the practice of gathering continued day after day, week after week, year after year, we felt ourselves truly becoming one. Not compartmentalized but integrated. I slowly but certainly matured and came to love my whole self. My heart and life began to expand as I became fundamentally more loving and inclusive, making space in my life for anyone and everyone who crossed my path. For we can only love others to the extent that we love and accept ourselves. Our whole selves. Even the parts we don't like. Know thyself. RIP Socrates.*

When you put in the hard work of being present to yourself, you notice yourself becoming more comfortable in your own skin. You feel less angst and fear. You no longer have anything to gain or lose or prove, so arguing with others becomes a futile and boring pursuit. Internal peace extends outward so you're able to rest in peace during life's storms. You still get battered and hurt, but the storms can no longer destroy your soul. You finally understand that you are enough. Now, and only now, do you have something of value to offer the world: your presence and your soul. Now you can truly be wherever you are, your whole self, occupying one space in one place. You're free to listen to others with empathy and sympathy and kindness and grace—without judgment. And just as the squirrel is content being, and the great oak is content being, so now you are content being.

Presence is the point. For you can only experience love and life and the sacred in the moment right now. One place. One space.

Upon my ALS diagnosis at the age of forty-three, I knew what I was facing. A shorter life with a disease that would first strip me of all my human functions and then kill me. It would take my ability to walk and use my arms. It would slowly kill my use of all voluntary muscles. It would take away my ability to eat and speak, and eventually my ability to breathe. I've said this before, but it's worth repeating: As the symptoms began to plague my body, I realized I was made for this. For years I'd been practicing how to sit alone in sacred silence. I'd been practicing talking less and listening more. I'd been practicing living in the present.

ALS even has a built-in presence reminder just in case I forget. Because I can't move myself, I get uncomfortable; crazily enough, my elbows often hurt and need pressure relief. A tip should you choose the path of practicing presence: Whenever you find yourself drifting out of the moment, simply ask yourself, *How do my elbows feel?* Then come back to your life, in this place and space. And experience it now.

Life is a beautiful clusterfuck and love is here.
Onward. Forward.*
love.

CHAPTER 10

ALS III

> *"Ain't no trouble gonna get to me,*
> *Nobody's gon bring me down,*
> *No worries will come to my mind,*
> *I'm standing on higher ground."*
> —Anders Osborne; Higher Ground

I'd already lost so much as I entered year three of ALS, and now the stage of the disease I feared the most was here: the loss of my voice. More than losing my ability to eat, or even the ability to breathe on my own in the future, losing the ability to speak was my greatest fear. In many ways I felt my voice was my greatest gift. To no longer have my own voice with which to talk to my wife and kids, and for them to no longer be able to hear my voice say "I love you"—this was soul-crushing and the cause of countless tears for me.

My custom since being diagnosed was to record monthly updates and upload them to YouTube. May 2022 marked the first time I spoke an update using my eyes and my computer. I could still make sounds and squeeze out little words, but my conversational days were over. I felt sad. In May, I journaled,

> *My voice is escaping me quickly. It's so weak, I pretty much whisper and hope they can read my lips. It is going away. Forever. And I can't help but cry about it. This is heart-wrenching. This feels like you're being gutted. This hits you in depths you didn't even know you had. This feels like your heart is being broken into*

a million pieces, that kind of sadness. It hurts. They don't make medicine for this. This is simply a path you have to walk. There are no shortcuts for this.

And yet, in the same month I also journaled,

When I think about my life, I still can't personally wrap my head around how we got here. And yet, at the same time, in so many ways, I feel like I fell out of the lucky tree, hitting every branch on the way down, and then landed in a pool filled with cash and Sour Patch Kids.* What an interesting life.

That has always been my ALS experience: really good days and really bad ones. The truth is, however, if I were to add them up and compare totals, the good days would win. As I've said before, my life is a living, breathing juxtaposition.

One advantage to having my computer working with my eyes was being able to journal again. My video updates had been serving as my journal entries for the previous year and a half, but I was only recording those once a month. I could now get back to actual journaling, a practice I began in 1999.

With my voice all but gone, ALS had only two things left to steal from me: my breath and my life. For most people with ALS, these losses happen at the same time, as up to 95 percent of people with this disease choose not to get trached and live on a ventilator. The reasons are threefold. It's incredibly expensive. It's very taxing on loved ones. And finally, living with ALS might be one of the most difficult ways to exist in this world.

Kristy and I had already decided that when the time came, I would get a tracheotomy. We weren't sure in the early stages of the disease, but as the disease progressed, I felt up to the challenge, as did Kristy. The good news as year two turned into three was that my lungs were still strong, and I felt strong too. In year three, I began to have eyes to see just how beautiful a gift ALS had been to me. My kids were getting older; I now had four teenage boys. Our conversations were becoming deeper, more genuine and real. In June 2022, we officially started the Diamond Dogs* and began meeting as a group on Sunday nights. We would sit together in my bedroom and one by one check in, telling the group what was going on in our lives. What was really going on—no one got a pass to just say, "I'm good." After each Dog spoke, we sat in silence and held their story in our hearts. After check-in, we each asked a question. Everyone had to ask a question, and everyone had to be asked. This has been our practice for years now, as we continue to develop deeper relationships with and love for one another.

In addition, I started a weekly get-together with Zoe Moon called Three Questions, during which we take about thirty minutes to ask each other three questions about anything. She was only eleven when we began this practice, so her questions were a bit awkward. One of her first questions was, "Do you like having ALS?" To which I responded, "I don't like having ALS, but I am grateful for some of the things it has given to me, like being able to spend more time with you." As time progressed, we made it to deeper and more important questions, and now our relationship is really growing.

By August 2022, my nighttime routine was becoming more difficult, as were the nights themselves. Getting me prepped and in bed ready to sleep easily took an hour, and often three people. By this time, I was unable to take a deep enough breath to cough mucus up, and I couldn't swallow well either, which made what had become major saliva production impossible to manage on my own. Both my inability to cough stuff up and my inability to swallow saliva were signs that trach time was near. I was still breathing well, though, so we were hoping to put off the ventilator until early 2023.

August was also the last time I uttered words with my mouth. I made sure my last words were "I love you" to Kristy and the kids, and I closed out with the final word simply being,

love.

In September, our mutual birthday month, Kristy planned an epic girls' trip to New York City for us. We would see six shows in four days. The theatre has always been one of my absolute favorite outings. Upon my diagnosis, my parents gave us lifelong season tickets to the Saenger, New Orleans's most beautiful theatre, built in 1927. Along to New York with us came our son, Micah, and three friends: Liz, aka E-dizzle; Andrea, aka Andrea; and Emmily, aka E Milli. I told Micah our sole purpose as the two guys on this trip was to be eye candy.

Dr. Kantrow was incredibly nervous about our travel plan, but we felt confident and at peace, so we took to the air. We hadn't flown in quite a while, and this was my first time flying while completely paralyzed. It was quite an experience. Airlines don't make it particularly easy for paralyzed people to fly, so we improvised, first rolling me in my chair down the gateway to the door of the plane. At this point, Kristy picked me up out of my chair and carried me to my seat while Micah tried to support her from behind. It took a while for Micah and Kristy to get me comfortable in the airplane seat, but we did it in time for takeoff. I sat in the middle seat with Micah on my left and Kristy on my right to balance me and keep me from falling over. Emmily and Andrea sat behind us with the cough assist and suction. They also supported my head from behind.

I was okay for the first half of the flight, but when my tailbone began to hurt, Kristy had to sit on the floor and push while the other girls pulled me up from behind. Kristy then finished the flight on the floor wedged between me and the wall to keep me from sliding down in my seat. In New York, we stayed at a hotel in Times Square so we could walk everywhere. We lived it up for four days straight. On our return home, my salivating and coughing kicked up a notch.

ALS III

I needed suction and cough assist more often throughout the day, and also at night, which meant I woke Kristy up three, four, sometimes five times. My breathing was still okay, but the coughing was annoying.

I could tell Kristy was worn out. Two and a half years of taking care of me by herself. Waking throughout the night, picking me up for transfers, bathing me, wiping my butt, feeding me, brushing my teeth, shaving me, and tending to my every other need. All of this in addition to managing the five kids and assuming the responsibilities I once took care of. Tending to the house, paying the bills, taking over the budget, taking over maintenance of the cars, figuring out insurance as we yearly added new drivers, dealing with the Sewerage and Water Board of New Orleans, and a million other things. (In New Orleans, having to "deal" with the water board is real. This municipality is such a mess that no one puts their water bill on autopay—because people have been known to all of a sudden have a bill for $700 for no reason. And yes, that's how we spell "sewerage.") She was exhausted, and I was sad and frustrated. Just as I realized something had to give, my friend and neighbor, Andy, called one day to say he was leaving his job and wondered if we could use any help. Within the week he was caring for me two days a week, and just like that Kristy had time to herself. Time for going to cafés, going to lunch with friends, working on projects she hadn't had time for. It was beautiful and felt like we had reached a place of reprieve.

We hit the jackpot with Andy too. We'd been neighbors (for seven years), but I should also mention that Andy is a comedian and part of an improv group and one of the funniest people I know. We spent most of our days laughing. And honestly, our relationship deepened as we began spending so much more time together.

In early October, we took a quick trip to Houston so Kristy and our friend Andrea could go to The Chicks concert and run the town. Micah and Lucas came along to hang out with me at the hotel.

Micah started feeling ill as soon as we arrived and wound up sleeping for most of our two-night stay. The first night I needed more cough assist and suction than normal. I continued to cough the next day while Kristy was out with Andrea, and as the day wandered on, Lucas wound up just sitting on the bed next to me to help. I, meanwhile, was also beginning to feel ill, which was nerve-wracking, so I stayed high to keep calm. Every hour or so I asked Lucas to put my joint in my mouth and light it so I could take two or three tokes. I was miserable but wouldn't let the boys text Kristy. This was her weekend. We were all asleep by the time she got back to the hotel. Lucas continued to help me all through that night and the next day, as my coughing was constant. Again, I stayed high the second day, but even so I began having trouble breathing. I didn't want Lucas to worry more than he already must have been, but I did have him hook me up to my bi-pap machine, which I usually only used at night for easier breathing. When Kristy got back to the hotel that second night, I felt like I had to tell her what had been going on. The night was rough, but we wrestled through it and headed home early the next morning, with me coughing the entire miserable ride to New Orleans.

Back in my own bed, I told Kristy I was scared and read her my journal entry from two nights earlier:

> *I am in a really dark place. I am legitimately scared for the first time. I am fearful. Episodes like Thursday night and last night and this morning, I literally feel like this could be it. Because I can't breathe, and then I start sweating and I think I have a panic attack. And it's dark. This morning, I felt like tapping out and that scares me.*

Kristy pulled up a chair next to my bed and watched me all night, administering cough assist multiple times per hour.

The next morning at six o'clock, Kristy texted Dr. Kantrow. "Call an ambulance and I will meet you at the hospital," he texted back. Kristy called the kids down and explained what was going on; they all jumped into action to get me dressed as Kristy packed bags. When the EMTs arrived, they realized they couldn't maneuver the gurney around the steps and railings of our front porch to get me out of the house. They had to put me in my chair and down the lift. From there they put me on the gurney and into the ambulance as my friends and neighbors gathered around supportively.

I was legitimately scared, which was uncharacteristic of me. I'd never been in an ambulance, I was gasping for air and sweating, and the EMTs knew very little about ALS. I remember wondering if I would ever return to our home in the heart of New Orleans. Had I just told my kids that I loved them for the last time? As I stared at the ceiling of the ambulance and the two medics—one male, one female—worked on me and asked me questions I couldn't answer, I just wondered. The entire situation was so incredibly scary for me that I had to ask Kristy while writing this chapter whether she was in the ambulance with me. I couldn't remember. She was.

After they stabilized me in the ER, I was admitted to the ICU. The next day, one of the most beautiful humans I've ever met, Dr. Kantrow, sat next to my bed and said, "Brian, we are at decision-making time. We can either make you comfortable as you transition from this life to whatever is next, or we can do a tracheotomy, which will enable you to live the rest of your life on life support. It will be difficult and very expensive, but you will still be here with us."

Sound like a no-brainer? Who wouldn't choose to live? The truth is, up to 95 percent of ALS patients decide not to get trached. It's an extremely challenging way to live: You're a fully cognizant human being incapable of doing anything except thinking. When my doctor asked me to make this literal life-or-death decision and I was hopped up on all kinds of drugs and still so scared from the day before, I was ready to die. But in the midst of all that pain and fear and chaos, I had a brief moment of clarity when I felt fully in tune with my wife, my own soul, and the Oneness. I whispered to myself, *Micah. Jonah. Nate. Lucas. Zoe Moon.*

Then, I looked into my amazing doctor's eyes and with confidence said, "I have a lot left to teach my kids, so do whatever you have to do to keep me here."

I woke up fourteen days later and asked Kristy when I would have my trach, to which she replied, "Baby, it's done. You're trached and you're back." This was the third and final undesired hole in my body, this one in my throat, completing the trifecta.

Apparently those fourteen days were traumatic. I'd unknowingly had the flu when I entered the hospital, and I came close to developing pneumonia. The whole thing took an enormous toll on my body and necessitated another twelve days in the ICU. Those twelve days were a living hell as doctors tried to regulate my drugs. I was on all kinds of pharmaceutical cocktails, which caused hallucinations; even worse, they greatly affected my eyes and vision, so I couldn't use my computer—which meant I couldn't communicate. I couldn't squeeze a hand or nod my head or point a finger. I was literally stuck inside myself, and hallucinating.

I remember one night when my mom was staying with me and I was convinced my night nurse was trying to kill me by overfeeding me and trying to explode my stomach. Every time the nurse came near me, I freaked out. But how does a man who can't move or talk freak out? My eyes would get huge, I would look at my mom with desperation, and I would cry. She had no idea how to help me. It was a living, wide-awake nightmare without end. I still don't like that nurse even though I now know she was only trying to care for me—that's how real it felt.

As the days progressed at a snail's pace, my drugs got regulated and the toxins slowly left my body. Then, on day twenty in the ICU,

October 31, 2022, our lives changed again forever. I was still pretty much out of it, but I have two vivid memories. First, I remember Emmily coming to stretch me. She entered the ICU room with these dangly Halloween earrings, and instead of calming meditation music, which was our usual practice, the playlist was Halloween music, and it was weird. I was in and out as she began stretching me until she got to my hamstrings—that's when I sprang to life and frantically typed, "I'm naked!" Emmily was one of the few people in my inner circle who hadn't seen everything, and I wanted to keep it that way.

The second thing I remember from that day, and what changed our lives forever, is the nurse on duty. I had some amazing nurses (I see you, Devan) during my twenty-six days in the ICU. I also had some not-so-amazing ones, and of course there was the psycho nurse who tried to kill me. But the one I remember best was one who cared for me only once, Mary Kate (MK). I was so in and out of it I don't remember specifics, but I do remember she wasn't out to kill me, and I remember how she brought peace and love with her every time she entered the room. Half asleep, I heard Kristy ask MK if she was interested in a side gig as a caregiver. Without missing a beat, MK said her contract with the hospital was almost over and she was very interested. You will never convince me the universe isn't benevolent, that the Oneness doesn't knit universes and animals and creation and human hearts together in love.

There was a lot of commotion that day. Dr. Kantrow was there, and the reps who delivered my permanent ventilator trained him and Kristy on it. Having only been cognizant for six days after two weeks unaware, I was regaining my bearings but still exhausted and drifting in and out of sleep. A few days later, Dr. Kantrow determined I no longer needed to be in the ICU. He wasn't ready for me to go home, however, so I was discharged and sent by ambulance to a place down the street called LTAC (long-term acute care). It was our understanding that LTAC was a place where we could practice home life under the supervision of nurses.

My room at LTAC was a nice change from the hospital, large and homey. It felt like the perfect place for practicing life with a ventilator. But then two nurses and a respiratory therapist entered and in the most obnoxious and unprofessional way started raising hell about how they needed to switch me from the ventilator I would live with to their ventilator. They proceeded to have a heated conversation in front of me and Kristy, who immediately got on the phone with Dr. Kantrow. He said he would get there as soon as he could, probably in a few hours. I looked at Kristy and in front of all the staff said, "Pack us up, we're getting the fuck out of here." I made sure my computer volume was nice and loud so it could be heard down the corridor.

I told them I would not be switching vents and they could discharge me. Fortunately, I'm married to my better half, who asked if I could stay on my vent just until our pulmonologist arrived. They acquiesced. As usual, Kristy won by being cool, calm, and collected. Once Dr. Kantrow arrived and explained the situation and how things were going to go down, everyone chilled out, and we stayed for four days.

When I rolled into our home after one month away, I was overcome with emotion and three thoughts:

1. How grateful I was for life.
2. How grateful I was for Kristy and my kids.
3. Fuck you, ALS, you mofo.

They rolled me straight to my room and put me in bed, and I slept for two weeks. Then it was time to get moving again. At that point I'd been in bed for six straight weeks. As we began this new era, life with a ventilator, everything was different. Transfers were different, as we started using a Hoyer (an electric lift). Showers were different. Going to the bathroom was different. Van rides were different. Stretching was different. The most difficult difference to adjust to was how I sat in my chair. Positions that had previously been comfortable weren't possible anymore, either because they would mess up the angle of my eye gaze, or because the location of the vent got in the way. In addition, I'd lost a tremendous amount of strength in my neck from muscle atrophy and was now hardly able to move my head. It felt like we were starting over, like nothing we'd done for the past two and a half years worked anymore. So, we did what we do as a family. We adapted.

One month after I came home from the hospital and LTAC, MK joined our family. Now we had two daily caregivers to help with everything from getting me up in the morning, assisting my bathroom routine, showering me, feeding me, giving me my medicine, administering cough assist and suction, helping me resituate in my chair—everything. While I worked on my own stuff, like this book, they did laundry, washed the dishes, ran to CVS, and whatever else it took to give Kristy and the kids reprieve from my disease. For eight to twelve hours a day, we now got to operate like a family whose dad was away at his job. In many ways, the caregivers brought a sense of normalcy to our lives. MK became a master at driving my chair, so she could take me to my regular coffee shop, and Andy became a master at driving the van, so I could now go back to City Park or the movies. That is the role of caregiver: to give the whole family reprieve. For the first time since my diagnosis, Kristy could be a wife and mom, and the kids could be kids again. Nothing could have made me happier for Kristy and the kids. The gift of simply being married again was wonderful. Kristy still took care of me at night and on weekends, but during the week she was free. This is what caregivers have continued to give our family.

As neither caregiver had worked at this level with ALS patients before, Kristy had to train them in all things Brian. The first time

Kristy trained MK on showering me, I was a bit uncomfortable and felt awkward. Before they took my computer away so it wouldn't get wet, I said to MK, "Before we get in the shower, I need to tell you about a condition I have that they probably didn't teach you about in nursing school. It's called Shrinky Dick, and it's what happens to a penis when it's not used for some time." She rolled with it, and I knew we had a keeper. When we got down to showering, you can imagine my excitement—if you're a straight male, that is—at the idea of showering with two beautiful women. All I have to say about that is that Porn Hub is a liar. It was nothing like that. Nothing. Moving on.

As for MK, she was one of the greatest gifts, not just to me but to our entire family. She's exactly what The Jeansonne 7 needed at that precise moment in our timeline. MK brought into our home and our family the same peace and love she'd brought into my hospital room weeks earlier. She invested her life into ours. She treated me like a king and cared for me as though we'd been lifelong friends. I did the math a million times, and every time the math revealed that I was old enough to be her dad. Now I had six kids—and the sixth was also my friend. The way she loved Kristy and the kids was special. MK put new systems in place for taking care of me, streamlining everything for future caregivers, as well as organizing supplies and working with Kristy to refine how we ordered medical supplies. She also began recruiting other nurses who she thought would be a good fit for our family. I would interview and hire them, and she would train them. We met MK on day twenty of twenty-six in the ICU. I can't imagine our life without MK had everything gone smoothly in the hospital and I'd been discharged earlier. Grateful is not a rich enough word to express the way this experience played out. Perhaps, love.

As I've said, life on the vent changed everything for us, and that includes parenting. I'd been home for about six weeks when one night Nate, fifteen at the time, asked, "Dad, could I go to Maddie's house for a party tonight? And Dad, I really want you to think long and hard before you answer because I can unplug you."

Other changes weren't so cute. For instance, I'd lost the ability to open my mouth, and I no longer had control of my tongue. I began having major issues with biting my tongue. Whenever I yawned, my tongue would slip out of my mouth, and when my jaw slammed shut on its own accord, my tongue became the unintended victim. My teeth almost severed it on more than one occasion. Besides the excruciating pain, I worried I wouldn't be able to talk if I bit off my tongue. Let that sink in, and then feel free to laugh. I eventually learned techniques to relax my jaw, which allowed my tongue to slowly slide back into my mouth, but it took months to learn that practice.

One afternoon Andy asked me what I missed most now that ALS had taken everything. I didn't have an answer right away, but later that night as I reflected, I journaled,

> *Now that ALS has taken away just about everything, the ability to move, eat, smell, and breathe, I have been reflecting on what I miss most.*
>
> *After discussing for an hour with my buddy Andy our favorite shrimp po-boys, roast beef po-boys, fried chicken, fried pickles, burgers, pizza, tacos, and more, for a minute I thought maybe eating is what I missed most. But then he stuck a vanilla formula in my feeding tube, and I got full and easily realized that is not what I miss most.*
>
> *At the time, I certainly thought losing my ability to speak was the most devastating loss, but as I got used to talking with my computer, though it was more challenging and time-consuming, I was okay with it.*
>
> *I have decided that the cruelest part of this disease is its robbing me of my ability to touch. To pet my pup, to hug my friends*

and my kiddos, to reach across the table to take my friend's hand as she grieves the most devastating loss. I miss shaking hands and patting people on the back.

I miss being able to reach out to my girl and hold her hand, I miss being able to hug her and wipe her tears. I miss coming up behind her and squeezing her as tight as I can, I miss being able to hold her in good times and shitty, I miss finding her body under the sheets, a hand or leg or foot or ass, just to know that she's still there. We are figuring out new ways, but I believe I will grieve this until my departure date.

This was a loss that would revisit me many, many times over the next weeks, months, and years. One night about two months after writing that journal entry, I had a complete meltdown and wailed for two hours. By this time, Kristy and I were sleeping in separate twin beds, and she pulled our beds together and held me. I remember telling her, "I wish we were just a normal couple and could get what we fucking wanted. This is total bullshit and unfair. I don't want to be a fucking inspiration. I want to be normal and be with you, even if we don't have shit."

This disease is a motherfucker, and though we were finding our groove, the pain of what we'd been robbed of was still overwhelming at times.

The trach did come with a few unexpected perks. I wasn't aware of this, but apparently all men in power chairs with trachs look the same. Suddenly everywhere we went I was mistaken for Steve Gleason. We would go places and people would shout, "Who Dat!" Others would ask for selfies. I didn't have the heart to tell most people that I wasn't him because they were so excited. But when I had time to actually type, I would explain that I am Gleve Steason.* It got so good that one year at Jazz Fest, as we tried to make our way to the front of the barricades to see Trombone Shorty, a security guard said, "Steve, y'all follow me." He then escorted us to the VIP section while hundreds in the crowd chanted, "Steve, Steve, Steve, Steve!" It was fantastic. A few minutes later, Steve joined us for the show, and I can only imagine what people thought. Will the real Steve Gleason please stand up?

By January 2023, MK had found a new caregiver to add to our team, a nurse named Britley whom MK had worked with in the trauma ICU. I just needed to interview her. We scheduled a time when they could come over together. It was immediately evident that Britley had an attractive and charismatic personality; she also had a depth to her, and an awareness of self that's unusual for most people in their twenties, and perhaps unusual for most people in general. She also had no filter and cursed more than I do. About halfway through our conversation I said, "Britley, you curse a lot. We really don't curse in this house." She turned as red as a Creole tomato. I could tell MK was waiting for me to say I was kidding, but I just let it hang for a minute. Finally, I typed, "I'm just fucking with you." I hired her on the spot. It didn't take long for us to jibe and for Britley to become part of our family too.

Early in Britley's time with us, I set up a meeting with the disciplinarian and the principal at Nathan's school because I believed Nathan had been mistreated by the disciplinarian. Nathan was the only one of our five kids who attended private school, and it was Catholic. Britley was working the day of the meeting and came along with Kristy and me. After the meeting, which went well, one of the administrative assistants asked to speak to Kristy. Britley and I continued walking with the disciplinarian toward the exit when suddenly the school bell rang and the halls filled with students. Britley lost control of the chair and ran me straight into a wall, exclaiming, "Oh shit!" right there in front of the Catholic schoolkids and the disciplinarian. This is how she came to be affectionately known as Oh Shit Brit, or OSB. Britley is even younger than MK is; now I had two new daughters.

In February of that year, I had the opportunity to meet Alanis Morissette. In order for this story to work, we need to rewind just a bit. The previous October, I had posted the following on Facebook:

I saw Alanis Morissette at Jazz Fest 2019. She was seven months pregnant and was singing her Jagged Little Pill *album. And it was great because it was Alanis Fucking Morissette. But it was missing something. This was the "been to hell and back" and came out on the other side with scars and a limp Alanis. This forty-five-year-old Alanis could sing the words, but she couldn't channel the rage of the young woman who wrote* Jagged Little Pill. *Why not? My guess is she had walked through it. And she felt every part of it. And she healed, and yes, there is still a scar but not a sting. Only love.*

I recently stumbled across her 2020 album Such Pretty Forks in the Road, *and it was written by the same person, only a reborn version. And then a friend introduced me to her 2022 release, a meditation album called* The Storm Before the Calm. *The calm does come for those who do the hard work during the storm. And sometimes that means just holding on for dear life.*

I've never really been taken by famous people, not since I was nine years old and mustered up the courage to walk up to the best kicker in the NFL, New Orleans Saints kicker Morten Anderson, in the local Pizza Hut to ask for his autograph, and he said, "Can't you see that I'm eating?" So, I'm not taken by fame. However, I am taken by story. So, if I could meet one person, I'd want to meet Alanis and have coffee on my porch with her. I could be way off, but I'd still like to know her journey.

So, if anyone has any connections...

I figured it couldn't hurt to throw it out to the universe. A few days later, a friend messaged me and said she had a friend whose band used to open for Alanis, and if we made a video, her friend would make sure it got to Alanis. A few weeks later, I messaged a buddy who's a video-making genius. Jon came over within days to shoot some footage, and a month later he sent me a four-minute video. I sent it to my friend, she sent it to her friend, and he sent it to Alanis's people. A few months later, we received a message from Alanis's people saying she was very excited to meet me. Could we schedule a Zoom hangout? In February 2023, Alanis and I Zoomed for two hours and nine minutes.

Alanis was everything I thought she would be, and more. I have no idea what it's like to be an international icon, but I figure in most cases it goes to a person's head. Alanis jumped on the call wearing no makeup and looking like she'd just finished family dinner. For the next two hours we had the most genuine, soulful conversation. We talked about story, journey, formation, spirituality, and more. I felt as though I were looking into a mirror. At the end of the conversation, which only ended because I was exhausted, we exchanged phone numbers so we could stay in touch.

Also in February, I was experiencing deep and devastating grief that I was unable to understand or work through, and I knew research on psilocybin had shown its ability to help unlock previously inaccessible parts of the brain, as well as help to form new pathways in the brain. We picked a day, and my friend Crispin came over to be my trip sitter. MK was also with me in case anything went wrong. We ground the dried mushrooms up and soaked them in lemon juice, a method known as lemon tek, and made a tea to put in my feeding tube. The experience was incredible and helped me regain focus and work through some grief hidden in the crevices of my mind. I later wrote about my experience.

A few days ago, I took a trip. Crispin went with me as my companion and chauffeur, and MK rode shotgun in case we ran into any trouble.

As we set out, I had no idea where we were off to. Things started off like a normal day. I got up early for my morning run. As I ran along Bayou St. John, it was a beautiful morning and I was cruising along at a smooth pace when I noticed a guy about a quarter of a mile ahead of me sitting along the edge of the bayou in one of those fancy power wheelchairs. As I got closer to him, I thought he looked familiar, and once I reached him, I realized he was me. I was the guy in the chair. I greeted me with compassion and love and ended my run early. From there we began to talk and decided to spend the day together. Healthy me began to drive wheelchair me through our life. Think Scrooge and the ghosts of Christmas past, present, and future.

We began by going to our wedding day, both of us standing in the crowd. Well, I stood, and I sat. And we enjoyed the ceremony as we both wept. The guy and girl getting married had no idea where the next twenty years would take them. Of course, we knew, and as we witnessed this union, we both wept, knowing what this couple would experience together. The joy. The heartache. The sorrow. The triumphs. The highs. The lows. But one thing we agreed on was that this marriage needed to happen even though these kids had no idea what was in store. The me in the wheelchair wept uncontrollably as Kristy read her vows, knowing that she would one day be challenged to actually follow through on those words in the most difficult of ways, all the while healthy me held my hand in silence and solidarity.

From there we made our way to 8709 27th Street, our first home. We watched outside as we brought our firstborn, Micah, home for the first time. This was the same home where we began to grow our family, as Jonah and Nate would spend their earliest years here too.

Our next stop was 38 Rhine Drive, the night that I held Kristy on the sofa in the den as she sobbed, unsure how we would *survive the arrival of Lucas in just a month's time. We watched as they held so tightly to one another. We knew just what a delight Lucas would be, but we were both moved to tears at the love we witnessed in this tender, sacred moment.*

Fast forward just two years, in that same den. I had a dance party with all four boys as Kristy recorded the celebration of their decision to adopt Zoe Moon from Ethiopia. There were no tears, we both laughed, as we were taken by the immense joy of the moment.

From there we traveled to Ethiopia and watched me hold our sweet Zoe Moon for the first time. It was at this moment that wheelchair-dependent me began to weep profusely, realizing that my sweet daughter would never have a memory of me as a walking, talking dad. This was more like a wailing from the depths of my soul. The pain was unbearable as the healthy version of myself cradled my head and held my hand. This has been one of the most difficult parts of my disease for me, realizing my kids, including Lucas and specifically Zoe Moon, will only ever remember me as sick. And this was the excruciating, heart-wrenching moment when I finally came to accept this reality.

Upon the acceptance of this truth, I was able to find immense joy and laughter over our next few stops, which included Diamond Dogs meetings, the kids' sporting events, Comic Cons, and all the places that bring the kids joy. Wheelchair me was overwhelmed with a sense of immense gratitude that I get to be here for it, and I was reminded that this is why I am still here. I also realized I had been distracted lately as to my purpose.

At present, I am working on a book as well as meeting with people in person and talking with so many online, and yet when the kids come around me, I allow myself to remain enmeshed in my computer instead of giving them my undivided attention. And honestly, there is nothing worse than being preoccupied, for when one is preoccupied, they are no longer present in body or soul, and I will not live another day not present. Especially to my reasons for being here. So, if the book doesn't get finished or I don't ever inspire another person, oh well. As long as my kids and my wife get all of me, then my life is lived exactly as I desire it to be.

Ultimately what I came to realize is that this might be the most difficult way to exist in the world, and yet I am the richest man in the world.

On March 1, 2023, Kristy and I celebrated our twenty-year anniversary. My original plan was to take her on an Alaskan cruise, but with ALS now in the picture I was unable to plan it. I did the next best thing and planned a trip down memory lane. I had MK scheduled for that day, and Nate skipped school so he could drive us around town. I was so excited I could hardly sleep the night before and just lay in my bed wide awake, not moving a muscle.

Our first stop was at one of our favorite breakfast spots, Ruby Slipper. From there we made our way to Coconut Beach Sand Volleyball Complex, where we'd begun dating. Coconut Beach had actually been destroyed in Hurricane Katrina in 2005 and turned into a pumping station. We got out of the van and took pictures in front of the pumping station.

For our next stop, I'd arranged for us to spend an hour at our wedding venue, Southern Oaks Plantation. When we arrived, staff greeted us and told us to take our time enjoying the grounds. We made our way to the front steps of the plantation, where we'd stood twenty years earlier, and I reiterated my vows. Kristy didn't know this, but I'd recorded my vows when I could still speak, so when I hit play on my computer that day my vows were read in my voice. This might have been the smoothest thing I've ever done in our relationship, right behind driving her to break up with her boyfriend. We then made our way inside to the dance floor, where they played our wedding song, "When I Fall in Love," by Celine Dion. Kristy sat on my lap as Nate wheeled us around the dance floor for the entirety of the song. We spoke no words but only gazed into one another's eyes.

From there we went to our first apartment, to our first house, to our second house, and finally to City Park, taking pictures together at each spot. I was unable to do a lot of things, but I was still capable of being romantic.

As my third year of ALS came to an end, I realized it had gone just like the previous two years. Lots of ups and downs. Lots of laughter and tears. There had been some differences. For starters the fear of death came to visit. Not the fear of dying, because I was not, nor am I now, afraid of dying. But this year as I gasped for air, I was afraid on multiple occasions that I might be leaving Kristy and the kids, and I wasn't ready.

Year three was also different in that I recognized more than during the previous two years what an incredible gift ALS had been to me and our family. My relationship with my kids was stronger than ever. I remember one Diamond Dogs meeting earlier in the year that spontaneously turned into a ninety-minute storytelling session. Somehow the boys stumbled into uncharted territory and started talking about how my disease was forming them in positive ways. Unreal. They know ALS means our time together will be shortened, and to hear them speak of their own formation in positive ways was awe-inspiring.

I felt more distanced and disconnected from Kristy in year three. I didn't know it as I was living it, but I noticed it in retrospect. Even given that, though, I felt more fulfilled than ever, and I thought our family was stronger than ever.

I began to imagine: If a healing man were to walk up to me and say, "Do you want to be healed?" I would ask, "Can I have the night to go home and talk to my family?" And if he were to insist, "No, I need your answer now," I would say, "No, ALS has given me more than it has taken away." I'll unpack this more in "ALS IV," because my thoughts about and attitude regarding ALS are a moving target, but this is how I felt at the close of year three.

During my third year of ALS, I was unable to sit on my porch as often as I was accustomed to doing because now someone had to sit with me in case I had a coughing fit or got swarmed by mosquitos. I had no quick way of calling for help anymore. In addition, my rhythms changed. For example, I was now starting my bedtime routine much earlier, at 7:00 p.m. I did, however, continue to soul-search. I spent much of year three continuing to search my inner life and investigating my understanding of relationships, conflict, raising kids, contentment, life, and love.

Life is a beautiful clusterfuck and love is here.
Onward. Forward.*
love.

CHAPTER 11

ON CONTENTMENT

*"I don't want to just keep up with him,
I want to be better than him."*
—Jamie Tartt*

I grew up in middle-class suburbia, and I don't recall ever wanting for anything. I do remember how my dad often said it's best to learn early not to try to keep up with the Joneses. Just declare the Joneses the winners, and live your life. This way, you can get on with it and avoid the rat race.

I followed my dad's advice until my high school years, when suddenly fashion became important to me. I wanted Z. Cavariccis and Girbaus and rayon shirts. Contentment, or lack thereof, became a true life-killer as my wants grew: more impressive athletic abilities, a better car, a bigger paycheck, a nicer neighborhood. I did get the most beautiful and amazing wife. Which was pretty cool. But everything else presented the struggle of comparison and wanting.

In my thirties, I stumbled upon a personality assessment tool called Enneagram that for the first time introduced me to various in-depth ideas about my personality type, including that mine is the type that experiences envy in times of unhealth. It was a lightbulb moment of realizing there isn't anything "wrong" with me. I just have a tendency toward envy, especially when I'm in an unhealthy place.

This was helpful information in my journey to contentment. Unfortunately for me, however, it wasn't until I was diagnosed with ALS that I finally started learning how to be truly content. So much of my inner training had prepared me for ALS, but though I'd been practicing, I hadn't learned contentment yet. I use the word "learn" because I don't believe contentment just spontaneously happens within us. I used to pray that I would become content, but I never consciously practiced contentment. I figured it would magically manifest itself. But that's no different from praying for money to pay the bills while not holding down a job. At some point we must take ownership of our lives and exert effort and practice and discipline. We must show up for class every single day, in every situation, and learn.

I tried for years to force myself to be content. Our house was tiny and cute, but I wanted bigger. Kristy's engagement ring was absolutely gorgeous, but I wished it were bigger. I was a good teacher, but I wanted to be the best. I didn't understand that being content was a learned practice, no different from learning patience or gratitude or how to swing a golf club. It takes time and effort, dedication and practice.

When I was diagnosed with ALS, I was given a golden opportunity to either learn contentment or to fight it. I didn't know this at the time of diagnosis, but the disease made sure I recognized the opportunity soon enough.

It began with walking. We live in a pedestrian-friendly part of the city, and pre-ALS I rarely drove my car. I biked or walked everywhere. My commutes were sacred times for me. I wasn't content to lose my ability to bike and walk. It was forced upon me, and I was angry. I wasn't aware of it at the time, but I began to practice contentment by giving ALS the middle finger and wheeling myself in my wheelchair to my favorite spots, specifically the eight blocks to my favorite coffee shop.

When my legs and core stopped working, troubles with sleeping really began to teach me that contentment is learned. All my life I'd been a side-sleeper, and for our entire marriage Kristy and I had been sleeping touchers. Bottom line: I never slept on my back. But once my legs and core quit, I could no longer roll onto my side; besides that, sleeping on my back became uncomfortable and difficult. It never crossed my mind at diagnosis that sleeping positions would become a problem. For months I woke Kristy up multiple times throughout the night to roll me from side to side. She never complained, not once. I knew, however, that sleeping on my back was my forever future, so I chose to start practicing. At no point did I choose to be content. There was no mind over matter because sleeping on my back was awful. When Kristy curled up on her side, I desperately wanted to move and get as comfortable as she looked. Even more than that, I wanted to be able to move my hand to touch her face or hand or leg or butt. It took me nine months, but practice fostered an ability to feel content sleeping on my back.

It was a breakthrough of magnificent proportions. I was truly content for the first time in my life. When I reflected on the experience of learning to be content sleeping on my back, I imagined I could replicate the learning process to every aspect of adapting to ALS, and to difficult aspects of life that aren't specific to ALS.

Next, I wrangled with my inability to ride my bike. I loved the day-to-day bike I'd used to get around town pre-ALS. Long after my legs stopped working, I still kept it in the house, where it took up space. I wouldn't let Kristy put it in the shed or any of the boys ride it. Looking back on it now, it seems crazy even to me, but I didn't want to let go of that part of my life. I wasn't ready to accept my new reality.

I also had a Quintana Roo racing bike I absolutely loved sitting in my dad's garage. I knew I could sell it for good money, but I wasn't ready to get rid of that bike either. For me, part of the process of learning contentment was learning to let go. Letting go—surrendering—is an intentional decision, and it was a necessary step in my quest for contentment. Eventually I told Kristy we could move the day-to-day bike to the shed, and I told Jonah he could ride it. I also asked my dad to take my racing bike in for maintenance, and then I sold it. It was difficult to let go of both bikes, and yet the act of releasing them brought with it a new sense of freedom and contentment. Ultimately, I chose to accept my new reality, which included no more biking, and accepting led me to a place of contentment. I was slowly learning.

Acceptance and letting go are themes that thread themselves throughout my ALS years, and every single time it's difficult. As time marches on, however, and I continue to practice, it does get easier.... Put a bookmark here. I don't want to jump too far ahead.

As I continued to learn contentment, I was faced with so many difficult truths. I watched other dads and moms coach my kids, a role that I'd always filled. The school where I taught PE hired a replacement PE teacher. The restaurants and coffee shops where I knew everyone by name continued operating. I was replaceable. I don't mean that in a woe-is-me way, but in a this-is-how-the-world-works way. It was like I'd died and everyone and life just continued. Only I hadn't died; I was there to watch it all unfold and continue without me. And I was supposed to learn contentment here? When my soul was crushed? If you don't learn to be content regarding circumstances that are out of your control, you'll live under a crushing weight for the rest of your life. How is one to do this though, practically speaking, to find contentment in impossible situations?

Practice.

Honesty.

Awareness.

Feeling it. All of it.

Commitment to learn.

Learning contentment is not for the faint of heart. As I was figuring out one day at a time, learning contentment was more difficult for me than learning patience, gratitude, poker, and golf. Hell, it was more difficult than learning to be a dad.

I had two choices. To show up every day for class and commit to the process, or not. I knew I would become a bitter victim if I didn't show up for class. So, I began with honesty and feeling it. I was sad. I was crushed. I was devastated. I allowed myself to admit to and feel all of it. I cried and I cursed and I pretended to shake my fist. I sat with those feelings and let them impact me as I validated them. And then I practiced releasing them, just as I had released my bikes.

Soon, I began to lose my autonomy—my right hand was dying, and I could no longer drive my own power chair. I'd learned to be content with so much by this point that I was able to spend less time mourning the loss of my autonomy. Contentment came more quickly. I was getting the hang of it.

And then, my voice. No loss comes suddenly with ALS. Each loss progresses over days and weeks and months until, one day, the next ability is gone. I suppose the disease is kind in this way. You have time to process your losses, as opposed to a sudden loss of ability of function, like breaking your neck in a biking accident and instantly becoming a quadriplegic.

I saw the loss of my voice coming for a year and a half, and I hated and feared it. I didn't want to communicate with my computer and a synthesized voice. Then the day arrived in August 2022. I spoke my last words with my mouth. And I was okay. It surprised me how well I handled it. But I'd been practicing and learning, and those lessons had added up. I'd learned to be content sleeping on my back. I'd learned contentment when my legs had died and I could no longer run or play ball with my kids or walk or ride my bike around town. I'd learned contentment when my hands had died and I could no longer write or play poker or participate in family games or feed myself. I'd learned to be content when I could no longer eat my favorite foods.

So, when my voice, the one thing I feared losing more than anything else, finally died, I was okay. Now I could honestly say I'd learned to be content in all things. Well, almost all things. There was still one hurdle to clear. It proved to be the most difficult hurdle in my entire life, and I hadn't even anticipated it. Kristy and I had been married for seventeen years when I was diagnosed. During those seventeen years, we loved touch. We held hands everywhere we went. We hugged and kissed and flirted all the time. And our sex life was incredible. During the first year of ALS, not much changed. Things got really difficult moving into year two, though.

I once read there are two types of people when it comes to sex: initiators, and those who need to be initiated upon. The two types usually end up together. I was the initiator in our relationship. Therefore, when I was no longer able to initiate, whether with a backrub or head rub or just by pressing my body against hers, our sex life changed overnight. Eighteen years of amazing sex, wild sex, intimate sex, just gone. Stolen.

We were at a crossroads, and I had no idea how to work through it. No one had prepared me for this cruel twist. Perhaps I should have seen it coming. ALS robs you of everything, except your mind, your eyes, and your penis. In many ways I wished my penis no longer worked. How was I to find contentment here?

Learning contentment in this area was my greatest challenge, in life and in ALS. What I did was begin to focus on our love and our relationship, and in this way I was able to slowly find contentment in new ways of expressing our love. The sexual desire never left, and I finally quit trying to squash the desire, as it's part of my biological makeup. Love and accept all parts of yourself, remember? Instead, I learned how to be content in the struggle; I realized my desires were part of me, but they were not me. Kristy and I didn't stop having sex altogether, but the way and frequency certainly changed.

Even more difficult than negotiating the loss of our robust sex life was coming to terms with my inability to simply hold her, to reach for her hand or rub her back. I ultimately decided I would never be content with this loss, but I have found a place of acceptance. And I'm okay with that. I've learned to be content in all things except in not being able to touch the love of my life. That seems like a reasonable boundary. Perfection was never the goal anyway. Just growth.

I wish I'd learned the secret of contentment earlier in my life. I didn't understand that contentment is a learned practice. Like I said, I thought contentment was something that just happened. But nothing of value in life just happens. All personal growth arises from showing up for class, taking notes, and then implementing what we learn in the everyday tug-of-war of life.

Contentment is one of the more difficult disciplines to learn, especially in a first world nation where the rat race is never-ending. But the rat race is a trap that keeps us running in endless circles. If we want to learn the way of contentment, we must commit. Declare the Joneses the winners, and learn day by day to surrender to your life as it is.

I would like to add one point as a way of concluding this chapter. For the past two years, I've been diving deeper into the mind, mindfulness, and consciousness. For centuries Buddhists have taught that it's possible to experience contentment and happiness and peace through mindfulness, meditation, and understanding consciousness. Some great contemporary teachers, like Sam Harris, Adyashanti, and others, still teach this today. And while I respect the Buddhist teachings, I haven't yet experienced contentment through mindfulness, meditation, or understanding consciousness. That being said, I think it's worth mentioning these practices also require learning. I've spent years on these concepts, and I'm pretty okay at them, but I still have a lot to learn. Perhaps I will experience contentment with more training .... Or maybe learning contentment and understanding mindfulness and consciousness are one and the same? For now I maintain, as I've written, that contentment must be learned. If I'm around in ten years, I may revise my thoughts, as I intend to continue learning and growing as long as I live. But for now I say: Continue to put one foot in front of the other, keep showing up for class, and commit to learning.

Life is a beautiful clusterfuck and love is here.
Onward. Forward.*
love.

CHAPTER 12

ON RELATIONSHIPS

> *"I thought being invulnerable would protect me, so I pushed people away for years, leading me directly to my greatest fear: Being alone."*
> —Rebecca Welton*

Relationships are beautiful and scary. It can take what feels like a lifetime to develop good friendships, and sadly those same friendships sometimes disintegrate in the blink of an eye. The patterns of past relationships tend to dictate how we approach relationships in the present. I'm no exception to this informal rule.

I had three childhood best friends, Andy, Todd, and Drew. Andy and I were inseparable from pre-K through third grade. At the end of third grade, his dad's employer transferred him to another location and Andy was gone. Todd and I became friends in first grade. We lived just four blocks from each other, and when we were old enough to do so unsupervised, we rode our bikes to each other's houses. Todd and I spent most of our time together in fourth and fifth grades. Then, at the end of fifth grade, Todd's dad was transferred and Todd was gone. Drew and I met in fourth grade. He was my best friend throughout fifth, sixth, and seventh grades. At the end of seventh grade, Drew's dad was transferred and Drew was gone.

When I was twenty-two, my closest friend and I were practically inseparable. It didn't stop us that he was married and I was single—he, his wife, and I spent tons of time together enjoying life and friendship. Then one day, out of the blue, my friends walked away. My life unexpectedly turned upside down. We no longer saw each other or even talked. No more late nights sitting around discussing life and philosophy and love and the future. Gone. I was destroyed. I didn't know how we'd gotten to this place, how or when we'd crossed each other. My takeaway from this and the prior three friends that had suddenly left me: If you let people get close, they will eventually leave. That's what people do. They leave.

When you come to this understanding at such a young age (and many people learn it sooner), it shapes you, it forms you, it drives how you approach relationships going forward. By my early twenties, I knew that to get close to people meant to lay my heart on the line and risk its being trampled. So, I learned to protect myself. I built walls—amazing, thick walls of masonry— around my heart of flesh. The goal was to keep people out because the pain of their leaving was too much to work through.

For the next decade or so, I bounced in and out of friendships, some superficial, some that started to grow deeper. Unfortunately, I see now, I subconsciously sabotaged the deeper friendships to protect myself. Even dating relationships were difficult for me, and I found committing to a romantic relationship almost impossible, including to Kristy in the beginning. As I've written, she stole my heart from first sight, but I wrestled internally for the entire year and a half we dated, nervous and unsure of every move. Why she stuck around is a mystery, like blackholes or why some people feed the toilet paper from the bottom and not over the top. But she did stick around. By early December 2002, I knew she was the one I wanted to spend the rest of my life with, so I met with her parents to ask for their blessing to marry their third-born. I asked them because I'm an old-fashioned romantic at heart, and because she was only nineteen years old. They said, "Yes, absolutely."

Choosing a ring was the easy part. Kristy's dad was a jeweler, and she'd been telling him for years what she wanted. I also knew how to stage the surprise. Kristy had a beautiful knockoff Fabergé egg that sat on the mantelpiece at her parents' home. I snagged the egg and got to refining the plan.

Step 1: Place the ring inside the egg.
Step 2: Go to midnight Christmas Eve service together.
Step 3: Head back to my apartment after the service and snuggle on the sofa in front of the fire.
Step 4: Wait for her to go to the bathroom.
Step 5: While she's in the bathroom, place the egg on the mantelpiece in my den, and be standing beside it when she returns from the bathroom.
Step 6: When she rounds the corner and notices me and the egg, take hold of the egg, get down on one knee, open the egg, reveal the ring, and ask her to marry me.
Step 7: She says yes, and we make out.
Step 8: Kristy calls her sister Becky to tell her the news. I've prearranged that her sister will be at their parents' house, along with Kristy's other siblings, aunts, and uncles, and her two best friends. Everyone hears the news together when Kristy calls.
Step 9: Kristy heads home to celebrate with her loved ones.

That's it. Nine simple steps. Only an idiot could mess it up. That night, I found the idiot. Everything was going according to plan, but somewhere between steps four and five there was a significant breakdown. As soon as I heard Kristy open the bathroom door to return to the den, I got scared, grabbed the egg, jumped back on the sofa, and stuffed the egg between the sofa cushions. Kristy walked to the sofa and lifted her dress just enough to straddle me, and we made out for the next half an hour. By this time it was 2:00 a.m., and she figured it was time to head home. I'd failed to propose, but there was a bigger problem: Her family and friends would be there waiting for her. I couldn't just let her walk into that situation without explanation.

"Before you leave, I have something I need to tell you ...," I began and then proceeded to confess I'd been planning to propose but got cold feet, and that everyone was at her parents' house to celebrate with her.

She heard me out, thought about it for a few moments, and then called Becky. When she got off the phone, she said, "I'm not going home. You're going to have to leave."

"But this is my apartment."

"I don't care. I'm sleeping here. You need to leave."

So, I packed a bag and headed to my parents' house. When I knocked on the door in the middle of the night and asked to sleep in my old room because the proposal hadn't panned out, Dad was annoyed. My parents loved Kristy. I had a slight oh-shit moment when he didn't open the door all the way, and I thought I might be sleeping in my car that night. Of course, this wasn't my first oh-shit moment of the night. But if Dad is anything, he's loving. He eventually opened the door, turned around, and went back to bed without a word. So, now I'm sleeping in my childhood bedroom and the most beautiful and amazing girl in the world is sleeping at my apartment with her sister.

I tossed and turned for four hours until finally texting Becky to gauge the temperature. To my surprise, Becky said it had been an emotional night but that Kristy was ecstatic that I'd even considered proposing. I might still get a "yes" if I asked now. I made it to my apartment in less than fifteen minutes, got some coaching from Becky before entering, grabbed the egg, kneeled beside my bed where Kristy was lying on her belly, and asked her to marry me.

That evening my dad called me and asked if I would like for him to come over and marry us so I wouldn't have time to back out. I had jumped this one hurdle; I could wait for the wedding, which was only two months away. That doesn't mean I'd overcome all my relationship hang-ups. I still had a ways to go.

In 2010, when our boys were five, four, three, and eighteen months, Kristy and I began the process of adopting Zoe Moon. We knew very little about international adoption at the start, but we sensed a stirring deep in our souls to pursue the idea, and the stirring grew in intensity as time passed. At one point, we asked four of our closest friends and our parents for their input and thoughts. They all supported the idea. Learning that the people closest to us agreed that international adoption was the right pathway for our family, we jumped in with both feet—researching online, calculating the cost, making a timeline, and so on. We quickly learned there are adoption communities all around the US filled with people just like us. Kristy joined Internet groups populated by these people, and they began to teach her the ins and outs of international adoption.

As soon as we made the final decision to adopt, Kristy wanted to share our story with more people. One idea she'd gotten from her online adoption world is that many people make T-shirts to share with friends and family to raise awareness about orphan care and, more importantly, to engage loved ones in their adoption journey. Kristy was eager to do the same, but I wanted nothing to do with it. We had our parents and four friends in our corner. I was content with that. The more people we invited in, the more opinions we would get, the more emotional energy it would take, the more heartache we would suffer when they disagreed with us or disappointed us in some way. I'd been down that road before. I convinced her to keep it right here, in our safe place, with just a few insiders. (I was pastoring during these years and in that capacity had wonderful connections with people. But I only let them into my life beyond the church to a limited degree.)

The road to adoption was an amazingly beautiful one to travel. Every step of the way—as we saved money and found ways to engage our sons in the process—Kristy and I experienced overwhelming love and joy in our hearts and lives. We studied up on Ethiopia, ate Ethiopian food, and celebrated Zoe Moon Day on the twenty-fourth of every month (the day we submitted our adoption dossier) by eating ice cream together as a family and anticipating her homecoming. We kept it close to the vest, just as I thought we should.

Then, one afternoon as I sat at my desk at work, Kristy called. "I'm sending you a video," she said. "I know you're not into this stuff, but it's about a family from Tennessee and their journey to adopting their son from Ethiopia. Would you please watch it?"

I had no idea what an "adoption video" was, so I had no reason not to watch it. I sat at my desk and watched the chronicling of this family's entire adoption process, from getting fingerprinted, to completing their dossier, to flying to Ethiopia, to bringing their son home—a twenty-four-month process compressed into seven minutes. As I sat there by myself with my office door closed, something happened inside me at the deepest level. I wept at the beauty and the love I witnessed. The video's climax is a shot of the family arriving at the airport back in the States with their new son. As the family walks down the hall in the airport, they're welcomed by sixty or so friends holding balloons and signs and kazoos and flowers. It's a party of the most beautiful kind right there in the airport. Everyone wearing their customized adoption T-shirts, everyone part of something bigger than themselves, everyone engaged in the changing of this boy's and this family's lives. The joy. The beauty. The vulnerability. The love. I couldn't control my crying.

I wrestled with myself as I wept. I wondered how many people would be at the airport when we arrived home with Zoe Moon. I answered my own question: No one would be at the airport because I wouldn't let anyone into our story, into my life.

Years of wall-building had protected my heart from the pain and the hurt that people inevitably inflict; at the same time, those walls were so good at deflecting hugs, words of affection, mercy, beauty, and love that they'd caused my heart to harden. In not letting anyone else in (besides my small inner circle), I'd gotten good at being alone. If I dared look beyond the walls, I could see people standing on the other side wanting to get in. Some even tried to scale the fortress, but to no success. The fortress could only be penetrated from the inside. If I wanted to let people in, I would have to kick the bricks down myself. That was a scary thought, and yet for the first time in more than a decade, I realized the greater fear was of what my life would become if I didn't figure out a way to begin letting people in again.

In that moment, sitting at my desk with tears and tissue and snot everywhere, desperately hoping no one would knock on the door, I changed my mind. I changed my mind about keeping people at arm's length. I changed my mind about never allowing myself to be hurt again. I changed my mind about the walls I'd built. I changed my mind about the T-shirts. And I started kicking.

Everything didn't immediately fall into place just because I'd made a decision. In fact, I had to work harder at and be more persistent in removing the stone blocks, one by one, than the subconscious effort it had taken to erect them. Still, there was a lightness to the removal process because love, not fear, was present, and love is the stronger force. I started with baby steps, first by writing a blog about our adoption journey and creating T-shirts for people to purchase. A friend designed the shirt, placing a heart where Ethiopia is located within a graphic of Africa, and we put all the proceeds toward the adoption. Next, we opened up our monthly ice cream celebration to other people, inviting them to join our family for another month of waiting. In addition to those adoption-specific steps, I began to allow a few friends to know me at a deeper level by talking to them about my struggles and my joys, my ups, and my downs.

For the first two years of opening up and allowing people in, I was forever looking over my shoulder, wondering which friend would be the next to sell me out, but I became increasingly comfortable with my newfound freedom—life without walls—as time went on.

The day we finally received that call that summoned us to Ethiopia to pick up our Zoe Moon, we had friends with whom to share the news and the joy. We had friends who were willing to care for our four boys while Kristy and I traveled across the globe. We had friends who thought about us, helped us, supported us, and cared for us. And when we stepped off the plane in New Orleans and walked through the airport with our baby girl, we encountered more than one hundred people holding signs and balloons, and wearing T-shirts, to welcome Zoe Moon and The Jeansonne 7 home. My heart was full, and I wasn't lonely.

Since I kicked down those walls in 2010, I've allowed people into my life who then let me down. Some people have ended friendships with me because I told them something that they didn't like. Some have left because I changed my mind about things we'd previously agreed on, and a few others have walked out of my life without explanation. One person who left was my closest friend for almost a decade. Each departure has caused excruciating pain, as much pain as I felt at twenty-two, but I understand now that pain is sometimes a natural consequence of opening yourself up to relationships.

So, how does a person get through the pain of relationships that end and continue to resist building walls to keep people out? As I've said in other parts of this book, I don't have easy recipes. I do, however, have my experience, and I have ALS, which has taught me a few things about both beautiful relationships and broken ones. As I've learned to keep myself from rebuilding walls, I've picked up some tools to use in relationships, including in the dissolution of relationships. What's come in most handy is knowing myself through soul work, paying attention to my inner life, and learning to love myself.

These days, when a friend leaves, or when a relationship breaks, I allow myself to feel the depths of the pain. It's heart-crushingly painful when a friend leaves; there's no way around it. So, I grieve the loss. Next, I search my soul for what part I might have played in the relationship's fracturing. One thing I've learned is relationships rarely break because of one person. I try to figure out the role I played in the fracturing (though this can be difficult if the other party won't talk about it). In the cases when relationships ended because, as I mentioned earlier, I changed my mind, the change of mind was regarding doctrines of the Christian religion—like when I came to accept homosexuality as a beautiful expression of love, and when I stopped believing in hell. In these cases, there was nothing I could do about our differences. I just had to come to terms with the losses.

On the other hand, in the cases when relationships were damaged because of something I said, and in cases when someone simply ghosted me—I could do something about those. I've extended invitations to several people to sit together and for me to hear them out regarding my part in our relationship's fracturing. To date none of my former friends have accepted my offer, but I'm still hopeful. Until and unless I hear back from them, there's nothing more I can do.

One of the many gifts of ALS is that I've been able to finally let go of offenses with ease. Unsure how long I might live, and with a prognosis of two to five years, I have no desire to harbor ill feelings toward anyone; nor do I desire to exert energy being resentful. Even as I write, I'm experiencing difficulty in a few relationships and I'm working on this chapter in a very raw place. I still refuse to waste any of my remaining days being angry.

When I could still sit on my front porch alone, I spent countless nights out there listening to "No Hard Feelings" by The Avett Brothers. This is my desire: to live with no hard feelings toward anyone or anything. Not knowing whether I'll be here tomorrow has given me the freedom to release others from their debts. I walk lightly, and when my body can't hold me anymore and it's time for me to go, I'll go with no hard feelings.

We only have two options when it comes to relationships: (1) We may choose to keep people out, which will certainly protect us from the heartache of people leaving and otherwise letting us down. Or (2) we may take a chance, place our bets on other people, all the while knowing we might experience pain at some point but also deep, genuine connection with others. I won't judge you if you choose the former, but I would be doing you a disservice if I didn't at least tell you from experience that choice number one will leave you lonely and alone. How do you do it, though, take such a risk? Well, you learn.

I have a friend I grew up with. We have memories dating back to first grade. As adults we stood in each other's weddings, and we even worked together. Then one day *I* ghosted *him*. I basically cut him out of my life. No more deep conversations. No more friendly banter. No more hanging out. I was insecure about some things and felt threatened by him, and in one of the greatest hypocrisies of my life, I did to him what had been done to me years earlier. He didn't understand, of course, and as time went on we tried to stay connected, but my heart and true friendship were no longer available to him. When I received my ALS diagnosis, this friend was one of the first to be by my side. He showed up on my doorstep with a cooler full of beer and two cigars, and he has come to hang out with me two days a month ever since. Reconciliation. Redemption. Friendship.

Throughout my time with ALS, I've experienced the most beautiful aspects of true friendship. Friends who sit with me, cry with me, laugh with me, curse with me, talk with me. Friends who are here for it, showing up day after day, week after week, month after month, year after year. Some of these are relationships I sabotaged in the past, but through tears and pain and suffering and conversation and remorse and forgiveness, we've reconciled and been restored.

There's another side to this relationship coin, and that's what we bring to the table in friendship. It's one thing to allow people into our lives and reap the rewards of their true, genuine friendship. It's a whole other thing to be given that sacred space in another person's life, to be one they allow in, someone to whom they make themselves vulnerable. What an incredible privilege and responsibility. To journey with another as they navigate the rivers and valleys and mountains and dark forests of their lives—and they with you. There's nothing more sacred and beautiful.

Perhaps my favorite master of words, David Whyte, writes on friendship in *Consolations: The Solace, Nourishment and Underlying Meaning of Everyday Words*:

> *A friend knows our difficulties and shadows and remains in sight, a companion to our vulnerabilities more than our triumphs, when we are under the strange illusion we do not need them. An undercurrent of real friendship is a blessing exactly because its elemental form is rediscovered again and again through understanding and mercy. All friendships of any length are based on a continued, mutual forgiveness. Without tolerance and mercy, all friendships die.*
>
> *In the course of the years, a close friendship will always reveal the shadow in the other as much as ourselves; to remain friends we must know the other and their difficulties, and even their sins, and encourage the best in them, not through critique but through addressing the better part of them, the leading creative edge of their incarnation, thus subtly discouraging what makes them smaller, less generous, less of themselves.*
>
> *But no matter the medicinal virtues of being a true friend or sustaining a long, close relationship with another, the ultimate touchstone of friendship is not improvement, neither of the other nor of the self: the ultimate touchstone is witness, the privilege of having been seen by someone and the equal privilege of being granted the sight of the essence of another, to have walked with*

them and to have believed in them, and sometimes just to have accompanied them for however brief a span, on a journey impossible to accomplish alone.

Witness. To know and be completely known by another. I can think of no greater gift in my life than the handful of friends who know everything and have allowed me to know everything. We love without judgment and without condition. I never would have experienced this exchange had I kept my heart behind that wall. All the heartache of broken relationships is worth the tradeoff of the life-giving friendships I have now.

Relationships are difficult and messy. There's always a risk of getting hurt, but there's no way to become the best version of yourself without the help and companionship of fellow sojourners. Relationships are where we learn selflessness, humility, and vulnerability. Relationships are where we experience forgiveness, redemption, and restoration. To lock our hearts away from others is to guarantee we will never learn to love or be loved.

Being trustworthy, honest, loyal, and loving—the work of a true friend—is a heavy responsibility, and the skills to execute that responsibility consistently take time to develop. I've been a fantastic friend, and I've fallen short as a friend. The bottom line: Relationships are hard, and if we really want to be in relationship with others, we have to do the work. The work will look different for each of us, and our work will differ relationship to relationship. For some of us the work will be learning to listen as much as we speak; for others it will mean allowing our friends to be where they are without judgment. In relationship with one friend, the work might mean tolerating their annoying partner; in relationship with another friend, it might mean opening your mind when you don't share the same parenting philosophies.

The really hard work, though, is your own internal work. Understanding what makes you tick and what ticks you off.

Understanding what your defense mechanisms are, and learning how to recognize them in the moment. Learning your reflexive MO in situations of conflict, and then learning a new way. Whatever your internal work, just know that at some point in every relationship, the honeymoon ends, the shit hits the fan, and when it does, you have a decision to make. You either jump ship or you learn.

In my experience, the more life has kicked you around and beat you up, the harder it is to be deep friends with those who have yet to be roughed up by life. This is what I mean by walking with a limp: getting roughed up by life, learning from it, and continuing onward with the scars showing. But true friendship is learning over years to sit in solidarity with another, whatever their life experience.

I think I was good in relationships overall until that night when my friend and his wife cut ties with twenty-two-year-old me. After that, unaware of the heavy baggage I was carrying around, I began building my heart wall, and it cost me a number of beautiful friendships. I became the type of friend I feared. This is why knowing self is so important. Until you know consciously how you've been shaped and formed, you're at a disadvantage in relationships and in life. If you find yourself in that place at present—either being an awful friend or suffering the offenses of an awful friend—perhaps today you can find a way to extend yourself, and them, a little more grace. Perhaps you could cut them some slack and allow them to be where they are, or lower your expectations to a level they're able to meet. It may mean laying down your ego and choosing them and their needs above yourself, at least for a while. That's really what relationships are, after all. Exercises in grace.

Life is a beautiful clusterfuck and love is here.
Onward. Forward.*
love.

CHAPTER 13

ON CONFLICT

"And in the end what's more important, being right or being kind?"
—Ted Lasso*

Conflict. The word alone makes most people's skin crawl. Conflict is neither fun nor enjoyable. It is, however, inevitable in any real relationship, whether between coworkers, friends, or partners. If you haven't experienced conflict in a relationship that matters, then that relationship is still in the honeymoon phase. There's nothing wrong with the honeymoon phase—ride that wave as long as you can—but in my experience, conflict fortifies relationships. Conflict may be the *only* way to fortify a relationship. I don't like conflict either, but after years of working on it and experiencing the beauty of relationships strengthened by conflict, I'm no longer afraid of it.

I've had my fair share of conflict, as you might expect from a pastor of twenty-two years whose entire job was working with people. It turns out other people are as complicated as I am. Unfortunately, most of what I've learned about conflict came from the school of hard knocks, meaning I did it wrong and learned the hard way, but that seems to be the way most of us learn.

Conflict's greatest source of fuel is that we all think we're on the right side. If we didn't all think we were right, there wouldn't be any conflict. Sometimes the first step to resolution is allowing the conflict time and space to breathe. Which, by the way, is something I don't like doing. In my experience, there are three types of people:

those who want to hash conflict out right away, those who want to sit with the conflict for a while before discussing it, and those who avoid conflict by running away.

I'm the first type. With the exception of times when I've instigated conflict (I've written about some of those times throughout the book), I don't like having any hard feelings between me and someone I care about. I worry myself sick if I sense discord. If you have a problem with me, or I with you, I want to sit down right away, for as long as it takes to come to some kind of resolution. As fate would have it, I married a girl who doesn't want to talk about things right away but instead needs time to think and process and circle back around to the conversation later. And it drives me nuts.

Early in our marriage Kristy and I experienced some typical newlywed turbulence, about everything from dishwasher-loading techniques to the amount of time I spent at work while she stayed home with two very young boys. We were obviously both feeling the tension, and finally we agreed we needed to talk. In my typical let's-get-into-it style of conflict resolution, I thought we might walk around the block to the neighborhood Mexican restaurant and talk over chicken chimichangas and margaritas. But she needed time to think about what she wanted to say and how she wanted to say it. So, we planned a weekend away at the beach to reconnect, recharge, and have some uncomfortable conversations. I already knew what *I* wanted to say and how *I* wanted to say it, but the beach was two weeks away. I had to wait.

During our weekend away, we planned plenty of fun, watched lots of movies, and built in time for talking. Prior to talking, we first laid out some ground rules:

- Only one person talks at a time.
- Once one person is done talking, the other then repeats back to them what they heard.

- We don't make excuses.
- We validate one another's feelings.
- We work toward a solution we can both live with.

It worked. Because we truly heard and validated each other, we felt rejuvenated and reconnected after our tough conversations. We left the beach ready to return home to our twenty-month-old and six-month-old sons.

These were the first of many uncomfortable conversations over the course of our marriage. But while conversations about conflict are still uncomfortable, we don't fear having them. We understand we're committed to each other, committed to fighting fair, committed to giving each other the benefit of the doubt, and committed to finding a win for us both. After twenty-plus years of practice, it often doesn't take us very long to work through problems anymore. Stay tuned, as I'll give you a little more about that in "ALS IV."

Of course, sometimes a conflict explodes before you have time to sit down for a conversation.

In 2008, Shawn was one of my closest friends. We got together every Thursday at four in the afternoon at the local Starbucks just to talk about whatever came up that day—anything from how the Saints beat the Bills again, to our dreams and hopes, to frustrations in our marriages, to poker strategies.

Shawn and I shared a passion for figuring out ways to come beside our brothers and sisters in different parts of the world and help them and their communities. Digging wells in Zambia, assisting new landowners to build homes with running water and electricity in Mexico, gutting homes after a hurricane rolled through the neighborhood surrounding our own church.

Back then my dad and I often talked about where we sensed the church being led (a larger leadership group was always involved in decision-making). Our conversations often involved my suggesting we hire Shawn to oversee our outreach efforts, both the ones in our own backyard and those on the other side of the globe. I went to bat for Shawn month after month until we hired him, and in the meantime, I worked to form partnerships with other churches and organizations that were already doing the kind of work we aspired to. By the time Shawn joined our team, everything was in place for our first outreach trip, to Zambia, the next month.

Technically, even though Shawn hadn't been on the job long, the trip was his to manage. I would be there for coaching and advising. Shawn was made for this work, which is why I'd advocated for him for so long; there was no reason not to hand over the reins. Oh, except that the trip was my baby, and I didn't want to let go of control.

Shawn and I spent seventeen days together in an eight-by-eight-foot room, sleeping beneath mosquito nets, without access to hot water. Add to those conditions a power struggle between two friends who'd never worked together in a professional setting, who both wanted to be in charge, and who both possessed strong, sometimes inflexible, personalities.

The tension was so thick that we were at each other for every word and movement. Then one night as we were climbing into our mosquito-netted beds, the top blew off. Relationship-destroying things were said on both sides. Fortunately, this friendship ran deep. We loved each other and were committed to working things out and working toward each other.

I asked Shawn for his recollection of the conflict, and he wrote:

> *It boiled down to control. You had been leading what international missions efforts we had and coordinated the opportunity to go to Zambia. Then I came on staff and wanted to lead, but you wouldn't let go, and I wasn't taking it well and honoring what you had done up to that point.*

After some bitching and moaning, we agreed that what mattered more was our friendship.

That conflict and our ability to compromise and come to a resolution forged an even tighter bond between us. We've had some disagreements since then, but conflict doesn't make either one of us nervous because we have a history of being able to work through our shit.

I'm sure there are entire books out there on resolving conflict. I've never read one, but I have studied active listening and engaging in healthy conversation extensively. My theories and conclusions in this chapter are based on that study, some techniques I picked up from my parents, and years of meeting with people in conflict in my role as pastor, oftentimes as a mediator.

Most of us are never taught how to fight fair or how to engage in healthy conflict. Instead, we learn how to handle conflict by example, usually by observing our parents. Kristy and I are no exception, and as our parents raised us very differently in this regard, we came to our marriage with different conflict resolution styles and expectations.

I was raised in a home where no one ever yelled. I don't remember my parents yelling at me, my sister, or each other, not once. Quite the opposite: My mom retreated from conflict to such an extent that she would go days, if not weeks, without talking to us. She was raised with the silent treatment herself. That's what she knew. (My mom eventually recognized this way of dealing with conflict as toxic and worked on it, so it's no longer her MO.) My dad, on the other hand, would spank me when I was young. He wasn't a great conversationalist besides saying "this is going to hurt me as much as you" before spanking me. Somewhere along the way he gained some new tools, and as I moved into my teenage years, my dad kept his cool when we disagreed. (I did not.) He always let me speak my piece and was usually willing to compromise. This is how I started learning healthy ways of engaging in conflict.

Kristy's upbringing was different. Here's how she describes it:

Growing up, I never learned how to handle conflict or communicate effectively. In our house when disagreements occurred, tempers flared, and the volume skyrocketed to yelling. As a result, I developed a strategy of avoiding conflict at all costs. Whenever the yelling began, I would shut down, run to my room, and attempt to become invisible. Fortunately, I don't struggle with anger, and screaming isn't part of my nature.

When I met Brian at the age of seventeen, I hadn't experienced much conflict outside my immediate family. Our dating life and initial married life were simple. After about six months of marriage, I found the need to discuss something that was bothering me about him. I thoughtfully considered my words, prepared what I needed to say, and braced myself for a heated argument filled with rage and defensiveness.

Sitting Brian down and looking directly at him, I expressed how a certain behavior of his made me feel. He remained silent, and my nervousness tied my stomach in knots. The silence felt overwhelming, and I braced myself mentally for the angry response I knew was on its way. To my surprise, he said, "I am sorry I made you feel that way, and I will change." I was dumbfounded and speechless. The conversation ended just like that. I had been ready for a fight, thinking that was the norm for handling conflicts. It might sound silly, but that was all I knew.

After the conversation, I called my friend Liz to share every detail. Repeating the exchange made me realize how easy it had been and how shocking that was for me. Could conflict really be this straightforward to handle? Can things truly be resolved this way?

Brian's ability to communicate and navigate conflicts has helped me grow as a person. I often jokingly tell him, "Thanks for finishing raising me." When we married, I was only nineteen, and he, having a few more years under his belt, helped me navigate life in a more loving way.

I have two couples in my life who've been married for more than fifty years. One of them is constantly at each other, bickering and annoyed. The other couple is gentle and kind, treating each other with love and compassion. The difference? One couple learned how to work through their conflicts over the past fifty years. The other did not.

Seeing as how most of us need some guidance with resolving conflict, I have some techniques to pass along that I hope will help you approach conflict and have uncomfortable conversations in healthier ways. Many of these ideas may seem like common sense. But if I've learned one thing, it's that sense isn't all that common.

Awareness

First, recognize your current style of resolving conflict. Awareness will set you on firm ground for change. When conflict arises, do you want to get into it right away like I do? Do you prefer to take a few days to gather your thoughts like Kristy does? Are you a runner? Do you avoid uncomfortable conversations at all costs? The first two approaches are acceptable ways to engage conflict. If you're a runner, however, and if you really want to experience fullness in your relationships, you'll want to make some changes. Lifelong runners will never experience the beautiful depths of true friendship and connection because conflict is integral to both.

Once you recognize your tendency, turn to learning some basic conversational skills, as well as developing active listening skills.

Active Listening

Active listening isn't just for conflict situations. It's the best way to engage in every conversation. Active listening is when one person talks without being interrupted while the other person devotes all their attention to listening. Here's the absolute hardest part for the listener: Listening doesn't include formulating your response or your next question or your witty comeback. Listening is *just* listening. Seems easy enough, right? Test your skills during your next conversation, even if it doesn't involve conflict. While the other person is talking, notice whether you're already preparing what you want to say next before they've finished. It's what most of us naturally do.

I've spent years developing the skill of active listening, and it's even easier to check myself now that I communicate with a computer. When I'm in conversation with someone and they're speaking, if I'm typing a response, then I'm not listening. My kids are especially good at calling me out when I fall short. They'll be in the middle of talking to me, and if they catch me typing my next thought, they'll ask, "Dad, are you listening?"

Repeat After Me

After you've actively listened and the other person is done speaking, now it's time to speak back to them what you heard them say. This way, they can confirm whether you understood what they tried to communicate, and you can ask for clarification if anything was lost in translation.

Keep at this back-and-forth dialogue until you both feel that you've been heard and understood. When you slow the conversation down in this manner and leave room for both sides to be heard and validated, working toward mutually agreeable solutions to conflict comes more naturally. Yes, this usually means compromise because that's how healthy relationships work.

Rules of Conversation

It's important to keep uncomfortable conversations civil.

No yelling.

No talking over the other person.

No name-calling. Come on, we're trying to be mature, right?

Time-outs are allowed. As a matter of fact, a time-out is recommended if someone feels close to losing their cool or just needs some relief.

The key to these conversations is approaching one another in love and coming with a soul open to hearing.

Decide in your heart before you begin talking to give the other person the benefit of the doubt. I cannot emphasize this rule enough. In straight talk, this means you think the best of them. You don't judge their motives as impure or malicious but instead trust that they're motivated from a place of love. A truly productive conversation requires open hearts on both sides. Yes, it's true that some people's motives don't originate from a place of love. Some people are just weasels, and if you're dealing with someone whose true character is a weasel, then you may decide to disregard this rule.

Practical Tips

Engage in conflict in person. It's a bad idea to engage in conflict through email or text for a number of reasons. For starters, it's nearly impossible to understand tone in digital conversations, especially through texts. In the absence of tone, we wind up reading digital messages from our own state of mind, often unfairly projecting our own biases onto what the other person has written and missing their actual intention.

Recently my nineteen-year-old son was arguing with a friend over text. They'd been going back and forth for days, and he was frustrated. I asked him whether he'd considered going to get pizza with his friend and having an in-person discussion. He said he hadn't considered doing that. Sometimes we hide behind our phones because it feels easier, but working through conflict face-to-face is preferable because you can more easily see and read facial expressions, tears, anger, and other body language.

I'm overwhelmed with gratitude for the technology that enables me to type with my eyes and the AI that has nearly replicated my voice. The technology hasn't yet, however, been able to figure out inflection. For someone who spent the entirety of his adult life talking to people for a living, not having the ability to inflect is a great source of frustration for me. No matter how I intend for the words to come out, no matter the posture of my heart when I type them, when I hit play the words are spoken by a computer in a monotone. At this point all I can do is trust that the people I'm speaking with know my character and will give me the benefit of the doubt.

Do not, under any circumstances, shoot off an angry text or email. (I've messed this one up too many times.) I know, in the moment it feels like this is the best email you've ever drafted, but here's the deal: If the email is truly that amazing, then it will still be good tomorrow once you've cooled down.

When Kristy and I were renovating our Midcity home, she found herself in regular turmoil with one of our subcontractors who was also a friend. She got a notebook for the sole purpose of writing raw, angry, unfiltered letters to our friend. She never sent them, but writing them allowed her to process her feelings and find the words she would need when it was time for a face-to-face conversation.

Don't enter into a conversation angry. Lay down your weapons of digs and slights. Even more importantly, lay down your agenda and come to the table looking for what you can learn. (I haven't mastered this tip. Far from it. This stuff is difficult in theory and even more difficult in practice.) When you truly care for the person you're engaging with, there's always something to learn. Don't show up to the conversation to win but to understand. This is the way for you to mature and grow, and it's also how to give your relationships the best chance for growth.

Some conflicts are too big for us to resolve on our own. If you find yourself at an impasse with another person, humble yourselves and bring in an unbiased third party to mediate—it could be a trusted friend, a pastor or priest, or a therapist. I especially encourage life partners who are struggling to get a therapist, as in intimate relationships it can be even more difficult to get out of our own way and to identify our own blind spots.

One warm night around one in the morning many Decembers ago, I was driving for Uber and encountered a fog like I'd never experienced before. New Orleans is sandwiched between Lake Pontchartrain and the Mississippi River, and on this particular evening, the cool waters of these two magnificent bodies mixed with the warm air. I was unable to see the hood of my car, and turning on my bright lights didn't improve my visibility. I picked up a couple in the French Quarter whose destination was their home in the suburbs about ten miles away. This trip would normally take about half an hour and net me roughly $18, but on this night it took me over an hour to get the couple home safely and I made $40 plus a very generous tip and it was not worth it at all. All I wanted that night was a guide, someone on my shoulder who knew the streets and could help me through the fog. Sometimes when the fog is too thick we need a guide, help navigating the unknown terrain of conflict. There are people who can help. You owe it to yourself and your relationship to at least try taking that extra step.

Sometimes, even when you practice these tips, relationships don't work out. Relationships do end, and sometimes that's the best resolution. It's possible, however, to handle the ending of a relationship in such a respectful and loving way—by practicing active listening and engaging in conflict with open hearts—that there's no lingering animosity. I know that might sound unrealistically optimistic, but I do believe it's possible to successfully end relationships with enough training. And love.

I've been practicing the approach to conflict outlined in this chapter for years. My closest friends are those with whom I've worked through conflict. As with all successful relationships forged in the fires of conflict, my friends and I have one very important thing in common: a desire to put in the hard work and move toward each other.

As I mentioned in "On Relationships," a few of my own relationships are still broken. I've undoubtedly had a hand in breaking each of them, although I'm not a mind-reader, and in all of my broken relationships I haven't been told what I did wrong. I haven't had the opportunity to practice active listening. Resolving conflict takes two willing parties. If one of the parties isn't willing to come to the table, no real work is possible.

I've failed at conflict resolution so many times, and yet, over the years, I've experienced more reconciliation than brokenness. There's nothing easy about this. It's much easier (in the short term) to run. But anything worth having is going to cost you. Like the relationship with self, relationships with others are hard work. Real, deep, genuine, grace-filled friendships can only be developed over time by experiencing the ups and downs and sticking with it.

It's my opinion that friendship is one of the most sacred gifts life affords us. There's nothing better than having at least one or two friends who know you, all of you. We must each decide whether the challenge of making and maintaining beautiful friendships—which by definition includes engaging in conflict resolution—is worth the time and effort. In my experience, if you choose to do the work, your heart and life will grow exponentially.

Life is a beautiful clusterfuck and love is here.
Onward. Forward.*
love.

CHAPTER 14

ON KIDS

> *"Most adults think kids need to
> be constantly entertained...
> Truth is they just wanna
> Feel like they're part of our lives."*
> —Roy Kent*

Raising kids is about as easy as putting IKEA furniture together. You never know if you're doing it right, and there are always leftover pieces. Also, once you struggle to the end of the indecipherable instructions, you almost always create something fun and whimsical and beautiful. Kids aren't furniture, though, and most hospitals forget to include an owner's manual. I've never even read a parenting book. Fortunately Kristy has, and she gives me the CliffsNotes.

This chapter is for everyone. It's for you even if you don't have kids. If you're an aunt or uncle or if you know a kid or if you ever were a kid. My aim is for everyone to find something to relate to and take away. Please note that this is the story of my parenting experience. I'm not saying my way is the correct way. I'm not trying to convince anyone of anything, mostly because at the time of this writing, my kids are still basically kids, ages eighteen, seventeen, sixteen, fourteen, and eleven. I have no idea how this whole experiment is going to play out. I sure hope I get to see our approach work out long-term, but I have no control over that. If the present is any kind of indicator of the future, however, this group is going to be just fine.

Part 1: Philosophy

If I weren't trying to stick to one-word chapter titles, I would've called this chapter "Roots and Wings," as that's our overarching parenting philosophy. We spend the first twelve years of our children's lives helping them develop a strong root system, one that goes deep and gives them a moral compass. From ages twelve to eighteen, we continue to help them grow roots as they develop wings so they may learn how to fly one day.

At age-appropriate times, we push them to use their wings, such as nudging them to resolve a conflict with a teacher or a coach on their own or allowing them to choose what they watch on their devices or pushing them to handle their own bullying situation before we step in (and I almost always step in until they are fifteen). They often fall straight to the ground before their wings are fully developed, and while it breaks my heart to see them in pain, they must learn to use their wings from trial and error. I won't always be here to pick them up. I can't give them their wings when I want them to fly; they have to grow those from their roots. The hope is that by the time they turn eighteen, their roots will run deep, and their wingspan will be wide.

This home and this relationship is the safest place in the universe. I'm your dad, and I love you. Whatever it is, I've got your back. I'm your biggest fan, and while you live with me, I'll give everything so you can eventually live your life without needing me. And down the road, if you ultimately like the way I lived life and parented you, you'll have a template. You'll make some tweaks if and when you become a parent—as it should be. Keep the good stuff and build on it. Leave the stuff that didn't work for you behind. That's what your mom and I did. We compared notes on the ways we were brought up. We kept what we thought was good and threw the rest out. Then we built on the good stuff so we could give the best versions of ourselves to you.

Our home is base. Homebase. Safe. Like in the game: When you touch base you become untouchable for the time being, so you can catch your breath and rest your legs before getting back into the game. That's our home and this family. Catch your breath and rest up before you go back out there. At the same time, our home is our training facility. This is where we train and practice. We practice how to treat others. We learn how to fight fair. We try on different clothes, and if something fits, we can feel good about wearing it on the larger stage of life.

When you think you're ready to integrate the word "fuck" into your vocabulary, let's try it out at home first because it's easy to mess up when experimenting with that word. It loses its potency when overused. Sometimes there's no better word, but timing and context are important.

When you think you're ready to get drunk with your friends, tell me beforehand and we'll weigh the risks and rewards together. I'd like to be the first person you get drunk with. That way I can walk you through it.

Home is where you learn manners and responsibility, and how to resolve conflict.

Home is safe. A refuge. Home is where we learn.

Here are some of the philosophical tenets that guide Kristy and me in raising our children.

Voice

This family is not a monarchy. There's no one walking around with a spanking stick.

Full disclosure: I was spanked as a child, so I thought that's what a parent was supposed to do. My oldest son got spanked three times, and my second son twice. There were two defining moments for me. First, one day at the mall my three-year-old was acting up, so I led him to the bathroom by the arm. The whole way there he cried and yelled, "Daddy, please don't hit me!"

The second defining moment was the time I entered my second son's bedroom to spank him, and he curled up crying in the corner of his bed. I could see fear in his eyes, and I remember thinking, *What am I doing?* I immediately talked to Kristy about it, and we decided no more. From that point on, everything was open for dialogue and negotiation, not corporal punishment.

I know a lot, but I don't know it all. There are two sides to every story, so you will always get to tell your side. I'm the safe place, never a place to fear. There are consequences to stepping outside the family guidelines, but even those consequences are negotiable. Everyone gets a voice.

One time when Nate was sixteen, he and Kristy got into a heated argument. Afterward, Nate came to me and said, "I didn't get to tell my side." Once they both calmed down, the three of us got together and Nate was given the floor. Kristy and I listened and realized we'd been in the wrong. We apologized, and Nate left the conversation feeling vindicated, valued, and loved.

Openness

No conversation is off-limits. No topic. Ever. You want to be a professional baseball player? Great. Let's talk about it whenever you want. I want to hear more. You think or know you're gay? Good by me. I'm always here to talk. I'd love to help you process and navigate those waters. You don't like the way I handled a situation? Let's talk. What can I learn? You want to smoke weed? Well, you're fifteen, and it's not great for your brain development at your age. But let's talk. As for sex, when you think you're ready, home is the place for discussing risk and reward. More than that, though, let's talk about how beautiful and sacred an act it can be. And let's see where your heart's at.

Nothing. Off-limits. Ever. And you can be whoever you want to be. Just be true to your soul. And as your dad I'll do my best to help you learn how to listen to your soul, as free as possible of indoctrination. Unfortunately, some indoctrination always sneaks in; as sensitive as I am to it, even I have blind spots, but I promise I'm always looking for them.

One evening the four boys got into a scuffle. I was already on edge when I called them to my room. I didn't give anyone a chance to talk and instead just started handing out punishments.

About an hour later, Jonah approached me. "Dad, can I talk to you?" "Sure, bud." Jonah then proceeded to tell me he didn't like the way I'd handled the situation and provided insights on how I could've handled it better. He was right, so I called all the boys back and apologized.

Trust

Trust is everything. I trust you until you lose it. And if you lose it, you can always regain it. The method of regaining it isn't correlated with time passing; it's correlated with a contrite heart. And I know you and your heart, so I'll know. With freedom comes responsibility, and I love nothing more than handing out new freedom. I love watching you mature and grow into the person you're going to be.

This is a big one in our house, especially as the kids grow older and have cars and parties and football games. One time one of the boys omitted a good bit of information about his plans for the evening. We found out and grounded him. The really devastating part for him was that he lost our trust. He regained it quickly because you can't fake that kind of remorse. He never lost it again.

Conversation

We will learn the art of healthy and difficult conversation. We won't shy away from hard conversations. We will learn how to actively listen.

You will never be made to apologize to anyone, not even to a sibling after you hit them, although you will learn the importance of the three words I am sorry. You will learn to take responsibility for your actions, and you will see remorse modeled, as I promise to always apologize when I've wronged you. And we'll learn all of this in the hundreds of hours we spend in conversation together.

At the age of thirteen, in his eighth-grade year, Lucas got a three-day home suspension for making an insensitive joke about a friend. This was the first suspension for any of our kids, and honestly if I'd had to put money on which kid would get the first suspension, I wouldn't have bet on Lucas. Here's the story in his words:

When I was suspended in eighth grade for some stupid words I said to a friend, instead of being angry at me, you talked to me and we came to an understanding. You did not make me feel outcast for what I did but instead you helped me, and we made a deal that I would not make that same mistake twice. This helped me build a connection with Eli, who is now my best friend. If it wasn't for the way you talked to me about my suspension, I would have felt too guilty to talk to Eli. Thanks to you I have one of the kindest friends there is.

Forgiveness

Forgiveness is key. When we say we forgive you, then we forgive you. Whatever wrong you committed won't be brought up in the future. There won't be any "You always ...," or "The last time you did this ...." And you will see forgiveness modeled in all relationships.

Nate, sixteen years old, was lying in bed with me as I worked on this chapter and precept. I read it aloud to him and asked whether he had any examples of experiencing forgiveness in his life with us. His answer: "I guess I could try to think of a time you forgave me and didn't bring it up again, but I don't really need an example. I mean, that's just who y'all are and what y'all do."

Respect

We treat each other and others with respect. If someone is a person, that's enough to earn our respect as a default; if they turn out to be a terrible person who then loses our respect, we grin and bear it, at least externally. While true respect must be earned, we live in a world where we must show social respect to certain people simply because of the position they hold. We show social respect to coaches and teachers. If someone wears a badge, we show social respect. You will develop a really strong bullshit meter and get good at identifying people who deserve your true respect and those who don't. You will learn how to recognize character in others.

This has always been a fun one in our family. Apparently not all adults treat kids the way we do ours. All five kids have butted up against this contradiction with teachers or coaches. The kids are so used to having a voice they tend to think all adults should be willing to hear them out. This has landed them all in the disciplinarian's office, which in turn has landed Kristy and me in the disciplinarian's office—and more often than not we're there to defend our kids. To date, our kids have been involved in the firing of four teachers, because in the end, these teachers were found by the administration to be at fault in dealings with our kids. (We never intended to get teachers fired, but to hold them accountable.)

Each time the kids have a run-in with an adult who hasn't shown them respect, I remind them they still need to be respectful. And they do it, but to a T all five of them fight for fairness and justice. They don't care how old you are or what your title is; they will show you respect, but they won't truly respect you unless you earn it. These kids have amazing bullshit meters. I think having a father with ALS has sharpened their ability to recognize sincerity, kindness, love, and compassion, and to smell a phony from a million miles away.

Rules

There are, of course, rules and guidelines and curfews and expected ways of operating in this family. Because that's how society works. And part of what we're trying to do here is help you grow into a person who doesn't live blindly by societal conventions but at least understands how society works and can function within it. We will learn how to follow the rules, and we will develop an ability to know which rules can be broken. Some rules can be, even need to be, bent or broken.

The legal drinking age is twenty-one, though I've never met a high-schooler who cared about that. As I mentioned earlier, I've told my kids I would like to be the first person they get drunk with when they think they're ready. I figure I'll get to see how they respond to being drunk and get ideas for how to coach them on future drinking. Nate thought his story would be a good example for how this precept plays out in our household. Here's Nate:

> *Drinking has its ups and downs. If I've learned anything, it's that bourbon is an acquired taste that I may never acquire, and that all the beer that Dad called junk over the years is actually great. I was fifteen when I'd been around enough kids drinking to want to try it myself, but unlike the parents of a lot of those kids, my dad's rule was that our first time being drunk should be with him. I picked a good weekend. (I was grounded for breaking curfew the previous weekend.) Mom went and got some of the drinks I asked for, someone poured bourbon into Dad's feeding tube. Micah joined shortly after when he discovered I wouldn't be finishing the twelve-pack. This wasn't free passage to get drunk every weekend, but it led to more open conversation.*

Instead of experiencing that for the first time without my parents knowing, and figuring out answers to my questions by myself, I had reliable resources who know me better than I know myself. On top of that, I gained a night I will never forget the first half of.

Third Way

We will learn that the world is not black-and-white, 1s and 0s, binary. There's always a third or a fourth or a fifth way of seeing things. Society likes to make everything black-and-white—or, in this country, red and blue. The truth is, however, that 97.6 percent of answers to all the world's questions are gray. So, when you come to me with a problem and you share with me the two options you're trying to decide between, I'll always ask you for a third option. Remember, there's always a third way.

When she was in second grade, Zoe Moon had a conflict with a girl in her class. I taught PE to this girl and could understand why Zoe Moon didn't like her. One afternoon as Zoe Moon and I discussed the girl while walking home from school, I asked her what she wanted to do about the situation. She said she either wanted to get all the other girls to dislike the girl, or she wanted to tell the girl how awful she was. I asked Zoe Moon whether there was a third option. She thought long and hard and then said, "I guess I could just try to get along with her." Third way.

Justice

We will learn to stand with the people society deems less than. We will practice generosity and learn how to stand with those who don't have allies. Life is hard. Always remember, it's hard for everyone, so always be on the lookout for those who have been dealt a worse hand than yours. And learn how to stand in solidarity with them.

During their elementary school years, all five kids went to the same New Orleans public school. Morris Jeff Community School integrates special needs children into mainstream classes. All five kids were asked by their teachers at some point to assist the special needs students or befriend a kid that wasn't fitting in, which fit our family philosophy.

The part of the city where we live has the poor on every corner. We've always made a practice of stopping to give them a few bucks or a sandwich; we ask their names, ask them what else they need or want, and shake their hands. Later, we seek people out at their preferred corners to give them what they said they needed or wanted. Sometimes it's a toothbrush or sunscreen. Our favorite, Sarah, always wanted a pineapple Big Shot soda. The kids really like these people. When we pass a corner whose regular is missing, they say something like, "Hey, I wonder where Jackie is today," or "Dad, I haven't seen Bongo in a while, have you?" (All of this still happens, though less frequently now that the kids are older and I'm less mobile.)

Soul

Your soul won't mislead you. Your essence is trustworthy. As you grow, we will teach you how to follow your soul and how to trust it. Many times over the course of your life, you'll come to a fork in the road and wonder which path to take. Your brain and your psyche may cause you to doubt yourself, but your soul won't misguide you.

Since the kids were small, whenever they've faced a decision, we've made pros and cons lists and helped them weigh their options. We always end the conversation by asking, "What's your gut, your soul, saying?" My oldest, Micah, is a comic book artist. He went to an art school for high school. The kind of school where the kids are a little weird, everyone thinks they're a progressive thinker, and everything is celebrated, especially individualism.

Except in Micah's case. He was the only comic book artist in the school, the most individual. And for four years he was made fun of for his art—my best guess is that the other kids just weren't into comic art, so they made fun of what they didn't understand. He wanted to quit his art so many times, but we always brought him back to, "What is your soul saying?" His soul always told him to keep going and ignore the haters, and at the age of eighteen, he published his first original comic, *The Stellar Sir Orleans*.

Risk

Life can be scary. You'll be invited outside your comfort zone. You'll feel trapped. And there will be times when you'll have to risk it all to be true to yourself. Risk it. You've got what it takes.

When he was around twelve years old, Jonah and I had a strained relationship. I didn't know how to fix it. I reached out to a family counselor and pitched the idea to Jonah to begin seeing the counselor together. He was adamantly opposed to the idea, mostly because he was scared his siblings would find out. I asked him to trust me and to take a chance on me. After about twelve weeks of counseling, we had new tools for connecting with each other. Taking the risk radically changed our relationship for the better.

Connection

We will learn how to connect with and know ourselves, as well as how to connect with others. We will also learn how to recognize that we're connected to something bigger than ourselves. Some people call it God, some call it Allah. Others describe it as energy or flow or consciousness. I call it Oneness, and I know I'm integrally connected to it. I will do my best to journey with you and teach you how to recognize this unbreakable connection in your own life. If along the way you come to believe it's just a fairy-tale belief, feel free to ditch it. But know that for me, I feel connected to something bigger than myself. My hope for you is that you'll find your home in the space of Oneness.

In Micah's words:

Growing up, God was never forced on me, but he was certainly mentioned a couple of times. Dad really would only talk about him whenever we asked him questions about it. But it was never like something good would happen to us and he'd sit us down and be like, "Make sure to thank God." He never pulled stuff like that ... thank God. It was just always said that we might feel a presence with us and around us, whether good or bad things were happening. Dad always talked of being in the present moment, and I feel like that was where I truly connected to whatever "God" was. It was him telling us to really enjoy a certain moment, or to step out of body and look at the situation and really learn to appreciate it.

Love

You will always know you're loved and that I'm proud of you because I will wear those words out on you. And I'm not proud of you because of your accomplishments. I'm proud of who you are as a person, a human being. What about your accomplishments? I'm happy with you for your accomplishments. But my being proud is about the person you are. My sons. My daughter. You never have to prove your worth. When you pour your heart and soul into something and see the payoff, then I'm overjoyed that all the hard work and grinding hours paid off. But if your hard work doesn't pay off, if you fall short, then I'm sad with you—but still proud of you for all of the hard work and grinding hours you poured in without giving up. My favorite thing in the world is when someone says, "Is that kid a Jeansonne?" To which I reply, "Yep, that kid is a Jeansonne."

Everything we do will be built on love. We will practice inclusion, kindness, gentleness, giving the benefit of the doubt, and above all else, love. If we indoctrinate you with anything, it will be this, for love is the greatest force in the world. Greater than any fist or curse or bomb. In our home love will always have the last word, and our desire is that it will have the last word in your life going forward.

One of my most painful memories is of when my boy, Jonah, was cut from the baseball team at age nine. The heartache is forever etched into my psyche. My heart hurt so bad for him. We cried together that night, and I reminded him how proud I was that he put himself out there and tried. He knew my affection wasn't contingent on any athletic accomplishments.

Part 2: Thoughts on Indoctrination

Fairly early on, Kristy and I felt solid in our decision to only indoctrinate our kids with love and acceptance—real, genuine acceptance, the kind that says "I see nothing in you that I need to be concerned with changing." Unless, of course, you're a serial killer or something. In that case, I would advocate for change.

This was a big deal for us, because at the time we made this decision I was still a Christian and a pastor, and I'd been indoctrinated myself, as I detailed in "On Journey." Kristy and I worked hard to buck the system that was in place to indoctrinate our kids, both at school and in the church. Very early on we began having conversations with our kids about the word "allegiance," and about how we only have one life, so we really need to think through how we want to spend it and to what/whom we want to devote it. We also discouraged our kids from getting baptized when all their ten-year-old friends were doing so, and we told them they didn't need to read their Bible every night just because their children's pastor (whom I supervised) said they should. What if instead we try Harry Potter (which is way less violent than the Old Testament)? It would actually take years for us to leave Christian traditions behind completely, but I've covered that story in other chapters.

So, if your goal is to not raise kids in two of the most powerfully ingrained worldviews your society deems good, noble even—Christianity and nationalism—then what's your moral compass for parenting? We decided to simply raise the best humans we could. I turned to my extensive study of Jesus, since I still think the stories of Jesus tell of a man who found the secret to a full, peace-filled, connected, and grounded life. I added to that the knowledge I'd gained from reading hundreds of books on relationships and love and interpersonal skills. And we also consulted our innate sense of what makes for a good human.

In short, we took the good stuff from how we were raised and left many of the ways we'd been indoctrinated behind. Our goal from the beginning was to raise our kids in a way that celebrates questions and burdens them with as little as possible to undo in the future.

Part 3: From Their Mouths

I thought it would be fun to get a pulse on how we're actually doing as parents. I texted the following questions to the kids. None of them had read this chapter yet. They didn't even know I was writing a chapter on kids, which makes their responses even more beautiful for me.

1. In what ways have Mom and I raised you that you are grateful for?
2. What have we taught you that you intend to carry through your life?

Here are their unfiltered thoughts.

Zoe Moon, age 11

1. Treat others the way I want to be treated.
2. You don't have to say everything you are thinking and don't be selfish and help others. Also treat people with respect.

Lucas, age 14

1. For me it is definitely that you have taught us it is safe to express ourselves. You guys have built a safe environment for us to talk about how we feel about any topic.
2. The thing I wish to carry on is having the thought process that everyone is struggling with their own stuff, so don't be like, "Well, it's worse for me," because for them what's going on is very hard.

Nate, age 16

1. I am grateful that nothing was ever off-limits. You never made us feel dumb or like we should not have said something in front of your friends or in general. And that any questions were and are always on the table, and you can feel any way about anything, but you can't treat anyone in a negative way because of your mood.
2. Something you have taught me that I will carry with me is that time and memories are more important than work or money. If I have kids this will be something I will try my hardest to do, and if not, I will use it up on a partner or friends.

Jonah, age 17

1. I am grateful that I was raised to talk through things with people. This helped create healthy friendships and relationships in my life.

2. You taught me to never burn bridges with people. This is something I will make sure I do for the rest of my life. We never know when someone may come back into play in our lives, so I hope I continue to never actually shove a person off.

Micah, age 18

1. I am grateful in every way. Lately, it feels we have seen eye to eye on everything, which I am grateful for. And that is due to your years of guidance. I told Mom the other day that if y'all were both to die, I feel that y'all have already prepared me enough for the world, and how to approach people and life in general.

Honestly, the question is difficult because there have been multiple times throughout my life where I didn't understand where decisions were coming from. Freshman year, I wasn't allowed to walk to a pizza place in a semi-dangerous setting at 7:30 p.m. at night. And I remember being pissed at the time. However, I look back now and I think obviously that was the right call ... because I was very stupid.

Sometimes, I wished some things were different ... like letting me watch "The Boys" before I was ready for that movie's gore and immorality.

I don't know how to explain my gratefulness because everything y'all have done has worked, and I wouldn't change it. Even though this new shit we're going through sucks, I'm at a place where I have been raised well enough to understand what's going on and can help in the best way possible.

Both you and Mom are still teaching me things every day.

2. You have taught me how to love. Even though I still struggle every day with that lesson, it's in my mind to continue it no matter what. Life is hard right now, and I'm okay with struggling with this lesson specifically, because I believe I have the

capability to get there. You taught me how to deal with bullies: don't throw the first punch, fighting doesn't "make you a man." I've also been taught how to respect women, but more importantly, everyone ... EVERYONE.

You have taught me how to talk about my feelings to a point where I am almost frustrated with how well you've helped me learn to read myself. Sometimes, I wish I could just be upset without knowing WHY I'm upset, but that's hardly the case.

You have taught me how to converse with people, and how to be with people. But most importantly, you've taught me how to LISTEN to people.

You taught me how to drive. I will use that for the rest of my life.

It feels impossible to express in words the things that you've taught me and how I will use them because I do them all the time. I feel like everything I do, I do because you showed me that way. So, putting it into words is difficult because it's simply how I live my life. I feel the best I can do to keep your legacy going is talk about you. Hopefully what you've taught me will reflect in how I carry out my life.

I have the most respect for you as a person, as my dad, and as one of my best friends. The way you carry out life now is how I want to carry out my life for forever. The way that you view the world is inspiring. The grasp you have on this concept/journey of life is sometimes frightening. Honestly, you remind me of Ted Lasso. You've given a lot. You always knew people's names, you always talked to everyone, you respected those who might not have been respected by the majority. Even today you do those things, even though life is not how we thought it would go.

Recently, life has felt like a fucking sinkhole that doesn't stop swallowing the good things. However, you've always said that you think the universe or the flow or the wind is a beautiful thing. Frankly, it's hard to disagree with you. I think one day I will agree with this, but where I'm at now, I'm just trying to get out of the "sinkhole." You just keep reminding me, no matter how bad it gets, it is still all good.

Part 4: Final Thoughts

I honestly was blown away by these responses. It's an amazing feeling to see the foundation we were inspired to lay bearing such gifts. They have strong roots, and they are now learning to fly. In the future, if the kids want to pursue nationalism or religion, or any other version of indoctrination that tries to tell them what to think, I feel they will have the tools to do so on their own terms.

So, kids, stay true to you. By doing so, you will be giving the best version of yourself to the world, and that is a gift the world needs. You are enough.

Life is a beautiful clusterfuck and love is here.
Onward. Forward.*
love.

CHAPTER 15

ON LIFE

> *"It may not work out how you think it will or how you hope it does. But believe me, it will all work out."*
> —Ted Lasso*

I started playing Texas Hold'em in my late twenties and was hooked. I watched and studied poker videos, played home games, and eventually made my way to the casino. One time at a $1, $3 no-limit table at the IP Casino in Biloxi, I was dealt 3, 8 offsuit—a terrible hand you don't play. (If you don't play cards, stick with me; the poker story is just a warm-up.) This guy across the table was incredibly cocky and had my number all night. I was on the button and had position.

As the action went around the table, everyone just limped in, including the guy who thought he had me figured out. One player raised it to $12; when it got to me, I made it $25. Everyone folded except my archnemesis, the original raiser, and me. The flop came with three spades, one of which was an ace. I had no spades, and I knew my archnemesis had paired his ace. He bet $25, the next player called, and I raised to $75. My archnemesis called while the other guy folded. The turn came, he bet $100, I called. The river came. Now, for all my opponent knew, I could have had a flush, a straight, or a set. I knew all he had were aces or two pair at best. The truth was, all I had was jack shit. He bet $200, and I came over the top and pushed all in with my final $600. He pondered for what seemed like hours and then folded. When I showed him my 3, 8 he lost his ever-loving mind. He went on tilt, and I took the rest of his money on the next hand with a full house.

What I love about poker is that you only get two cards, and you have to play those two cards. You don't get to trade them in if you don't like them. Poker, like life, is a game of strategy that takes finesse and courage and poise and luck and resolve. The difference is that, in poker, you can fold your hand. In life, you keep playing the cards you were dealt.

What *is* life? That's a big question that has kept philosophers and poets and pastors and artists and mystics and lovers of life and love, and me, awake at night. Searching. Inquiring. Investigating. Wondering. Asking. I don't claim to have cracked the code to understanding everything life encompasses; I have, however, stumbled upon a few truths that have helped me get closer to understanding what life is and how to best, well, live it.

To begin, let's acknowledge what a beautiful gift life is. We get to be on this planet that's billions of years old and, if we don't kill it, that will continue to exist for at least millions more. We got an invite to this global billion-year party. Imagine for a moment that a different sperm had won the race on the day of your conception. You wouldn't be reading this because there would be no you. But there *is* you. You get to pass a lifetime here. On the planet. You. Life is a privilege. Life is a gift. And you got a spot.

As far as we know, we only get this one life. Sure, maybe some of us have already taken a spin on this tiny blue-and-green ball that's hurling through space around a burning fireball. But I haven't met anyone with conscious memories from a previous life. What we can know is that we are here now. This is our shot. Which begs the questions: What will you do with it? Who will you be? What is the plot line?

Purpose

I spent the first thirty-three years of my life trying to figure out my purpose, praying that God would show it to me. Looking back, I see how much of life I missed out on while pursuing my purpose.

I suggest that life is to be lived, experienced, and enjoyed. I also suggest that everyone, regardless of individual circumstances, shares the same purpose(s): We're meant to live lightly and freely regardless of our lot in life. We're meant to be formed and transformed by life, to grow up so we may experience and offer the best version of ourselves to the world. Most of all, we're meant to learn love.

I'll never forget a woman I met while scouting places to build wells in Zambia. Her husband dead of AIDS, she was raising their seven children in a one-room mud hut. I remember her explaining to me which children got to eat today and which ones would be fed tomorrow. The circumstances of her life were heavy, and yet in many ways this woman seemed more content and internally at rest than I was. She lived lightly and freely, and she knew love.

Surrender

Worry, stress, and the need for control are thieves that will destroy a person's life, and the lives of the people around them. Best to recognize that you are in control of very little. You have no control over external forces. You don't even have control over what your next thought will be. Surrendering your life, and surrendering to your life, leads to experiencing your life in its rawest and most beautiful form.

Thanks to ALS, I now know what it is to surrender everything. I now understand the ancient wisdom that if you want to find your life, you must be willing to lose your life. Like everyone does, I knew I would die one day. However, upon receiving a death sentence in

2020 at the age of forty-three, I was suddenly faced with what true surrender looks and feels like. The surrender to a shortened life. I distinctly remember the pain of surrendering my hopes of growing old with Kristy. We had kids early and knew that by the time Zoe Moon was eighteen and ready to move out, we would only be fifty-three and forty-six years old. We thought we might move (Chicago or North Carolina or San Francisco), and I always imagined us growing old together, sitting in our rocking chairs, drinking our coffee, enjoying our kids and grandkids, and enjoying each other. That was a dream I had to surrender. It took me close to a year to let it go, but once I did I felt more alive and able to enjoy my relationship with Kristy here and now. I had lost the possibilities of what might be and was ushered into the present of what is. I had found my life.

In many ways, life does invite us to forge our own path; it gifts us the power of choice. Who do I want to love? What do I want to study? What type of pet do I want? What decisions can I make to ensure the love between me and my partner lasts until we're well into our eighties? How do I want to raise my children, and what do I want to instill in them?

We feel we have control over such things, and I suppose we do to some degree. That is, until others—people and institutions—exercise *their* power of choice. Sometimes the people we love don't love us back. Sometimes the school we have our heart set on rejects us. Sometimes on the day we finally decide we want a puppy the pet store is fresh out of puppies and only has cats left. In such cases, isn't surrendering the easy way out? Shouldn't we kick down the door? Win their heart with a grand romantic gesture; appeal the rejection letter and convince the university what an asset we'd be on their campus; and (please!) go to another pet store or to a rescue shelter that isn't out of dogs? (This is not a supernatural event trying to tell you that you need a cat. No, you don't need a cat!) Sometimes a door closing is the universe's way of communicating that you're not on a good path, but other times the planet hits a cosmic speed bump and doors all around the globe slam shut until you kick them down.

Every good story has a protagonist who must overcome some adversity to achieve a goal. They don't quit when the door closes. No, when the door closes, the protagonist kicks it down, or they find a window to crawl through. We love and cheer for the protagonist. Rocky Balboa. William Wallace. Martin Luther King Jr. Ted Lasso. Rey Skywalker. The Avengers. Nelson Mandela. Nemo's dad. We go to the movies and glue ourselves to television series and read good books to see how the protagonist will be set up to fail and then ultimately prevail. We're all the protagonists in our lives, and I agree it's sometimes appropriate to act like one.

But what if we eat well, exercise, and learn to love our partner how they want to be loved so we can go strong into our eighties together, but our partner decides to leave us anyway? What if we get a terminal illness in our forties? What if a drunk driver crosses the center line and kills our daughter in a head-on collision? How can we tell when to surrender and when it's time to act the protagonist in our own story? You know the refrain by now: It takes practice. Lots of practice.

A Singular Point of Control

Life is not either/or; it is always and forever both/and. Both amazing and awful. Harmony and havoc. Terrific and tragic. Beautiful and brutal. Calm and chaos. Victory and vices. Delightful and devastating. Love and loss. Sacred and sad. Epic and excruciating. Life is beautiful, and life is a clusterfuck. They're two sides of the same coin, and you don't get to choose which side is facing up.

There is one part of life over which we always have control, however, and that's what kind of person we want to be. This is a soul matter, where the treasure lies. We get to decide who we want to be, and then we get to devote our life to practicing becoming that person. If you want to be an asshat, then work hard at it. You'll get there. Your life will be miserable, and you'll be lonely, but you'll arrive at asshatness. If, on the other hand, you want to be a person of love and peace and forgiveness and mercy and grace and kindness, well, that takes more commitment and practice than the asshat route. Anyone can be an asshat; that's why there are so many of them. But love? That requires showing up for class every single day, including on the days you'd rather opt out. Especially on the days you'd rather opt out. As Friedrich Nietzsche once said, "The essential thing 'in heaven and earth' is ... that there should be a long obedience in the same direction; there thereby results, and has always resulted in the long run, something which has made life worth living."

A long obedience in the same direction.

Imagine two roads. The first road is wide and easy. The other is narrow and difficult. On the wide road there are very few consequences for anything. Nothing is asked of you on this path; you simply live out your life however you want. You follow your desires and don't question your qualms. On this road you hold grudges and withhold forgiveness. This is the destructive road of the selfish, the greedy, and the unaware, and so many are on it because of its ease, but also because they often haven't seen a beautiful alternative. It leads to a shallow place and leaves you and others in your life busted and bruised and beat up, but the journey is comfortable because you can avoid obstacles.

The narrow road is a more difficult choice. Traveling it requires discipline and steadfastness. You learn to practice selflessness and forgiveness along the way, peace instead of revenge, love instead of fuck you. You are held accountable for your decisions and movements on this road, which is often difficult and painful, but ultimately this road leads to greater freedom and love.

As we live our lives, we encounter many forks in the road where we may choose, again, which road to follow. When I was in my mid-thirties, I had a sense I might not be putting the person I actually wanted to be into the world. So, I drafted an email with four questions and sent it to two coworkers and two friends, asking them to answer the questions and promising I wouldn't hold their honesty against them. I needed their honesty if I was going to change. My questions were:

1. How do I come across to you as a person or friend?
2. How am I to work with and associate with?
3. Do you see me as a welcoming person?
4. Do you see any things in me that I may be blind to?

I asked them to write their replies and then meet with me and give me their answers over coffee. To my surprise, they all agreed to the plan, and they didn't hold back. It was brutal. I did not like the person they described. To a person, they perceived me as arrogant. Two of them expressed that I often seemed to think I was the most important person in the room. I recall one of them saying that menial tasks seemed beneath me, and another said I generally lacked love.

I gave myself a few days to cry, and then I got to work. I knew now that people weren't getting the version of me I wanted to be, so I set my sights on that person. I began taking an internal inventory on a regular basis, daily reflecting on my interactions with others and occasionally checking in with others on how I was doing. I practiced conflict resolution. I apologized. I surrendered parts of myself to a higher power. I practiced, I failed, and then I got up and practiced again. A long obedience in the same direction, day after day after day. Those were very challenging years, but the more I practiced, allowing my soul to be vulnerable and shown to the world, the more alive I felt. I also experienced more pain and difficulties in relationships. It turns out not everyone is comfortable with you when you finally choose to be true to yourself.

During this time of learning my truest self and enacting personal change, I brought in some friends I knew would keep the conversations gut-level honest with me. I'd met Crispin and Nathan when I was nineteen; they were trusted and safe friends on a similar journey, and they knew every card in my hand. I also picked up a soul care coach and a therapist. This was my team, the ones who walked with me as I looked under all the rocks and behind every door. They didn't push or pull; just walked with me. Except for a few times when they got in my face.

One day during a leadership team meeting at work, we learned one of our key players was leaving his position for reasons I thought were weak. I told Crispin, who worked there too, exactly how I felt, and Crispin asked me if I wanted to grab a cup of coffee. Once we got our drinks and settled into a cozy nook of the coffee house, Crispin said, "Brian, I don't know if I can do this anymore."

"Do what?" I asked.

"Be friends with you anymore. Your lack of empathy and your judgmentalism are toxic, and it's crushing my soul."

Crispin was one of my closest friends, so this hurt. "What can I do?" I asked.

"You can change," he said.

And that's what I did. I changed directions. I trusted Crispin. I felt secure in his love for me. I knew that conversation must have been difficult for him, but he had to take care of his own soul and life. It was one of those crossroads that you come to, and you don't have time to think. You have to make a split-second decision. I chose change. I chose the narrow road.

Around the same time, my therapist, whom I was paying, and to whom I was bearing my heart, said to me, "Brian, can I tell you what I think is really going on here? It's time for you to grow up. You're immature, and it's time to grow up and be an adult."

That's not easy for a thirty-six-year-old to hear. I left his office with smoke coming out of my ears, got into my car, and immediately called Nate. "Can you believe he told me to grow up?" I asked.

Silence.

"Nate, are you there?"

"Yeah. I'm here."

"Did you hear what I said?"

"Yeah. I heard you. It sounds like it was painful to hear."

Crickets.

Nate was neither confirming nor denying, which meant he was confirming. Fuuuuck! Again, I had a decision to make. Keep living in my bubble of unawareness or accept what others see in me and press into it.

Life happens to us all. Life is coming for you. There's no escaping it. Will you be life's victim, or will you be life's pupil? You get to decide. You've met your future self already. Will you be that crotchety old man or woman who's angry at the world and full of blame to pour out on anyone but themselves, or will you be the sweet and gentle and humble and kind and wise elder you met on the park bench the other day? People are who they are because of a lifetime of practice. There's no magic pill for who you are to become. It's a decision. You decide who you want to be, and then you practice a long obedience in the same direction. This is your life's work.

The Corridor

I once read a story about a couple who went to the hospital's maternity floor, walked the corridor, and found the room on the right where their youngest daughter had given birth to a beautiful baby girl, their first grandchild. Six months later they returned to the same hospital, to the same floor, same corridor, only this time they entered the room on the left. In this room their eldest daughter had given birth to a beautiful stillborn baby boy.

This corridor is where we live. We don't live in the room on the right; nor do we live in the room on the left. We live in the corridor between the two rooms. We so desperately want to live in the room on the right, but we must learn to live in the corridor with equanimity.

I grew up in a tradition of belief that every negative occurrence could be, and needed to be, remedied. If it was financial trouble, we prayed for provision. If it was an illness, we prayed for healing. And if it was death—I've been in a room more than once where people were praying to raise the dead from their sleep. Humans don't want pain or hurt, and that actually seems like a healthy reflex. Masochism isn't a positive trait. But in real life, shit breaks. And it can't be prayed back together.

It's by living all of it—the beautiful and the ugly—that we fully experience our humanity and can transform. Life is not a problem to be fixed but an experience to be lived. I just came up with that. I feel pretty good about it.* Everyone has days when they feel they can't go on. Those are the worst days. It takes everything in you, every grace available to you, to keep going. And please do. I promise beauty will rise from the ashes, likely in the most unexpected ways. To deny this fundamental precept of life is to rob ourselves of the full experience of life, her beauty and her brutality.

Humanity's greatest challenge is that, time and again, we expect life to be fair. Many people live with the belief that, "If I'm a good person, I should be spared from the chaos and pain." But why would anyone get a free ride? And, more importantly, if we were to be spared chaos and pain, how would we ever develop depth in our lives? Remember the both/and. Transformation and change rarely (never?) occur during the easy times. As I've said throughout this book, true soul work and transformation are born through great love and great suffering. Life is going to happen to all of us. Some will ignore it or try to will it away. Others will try to pray it away or positive-think their way out. It might look good on the outside, but there will never be transformation. Bottom line: It rains on the good and the bad. The sun shines on those who deserve it and those who don't. There is no way around it; the only way is through it.

Five Not-So-Easy Steps

So, that's it? I just decide who I want to be and, poof, I'm a good person? Unfortunately, it takes a little more deliberate action than that. I've never met a single person who completed transformational work through sheer willpower. No, there are a few non-negotiables, and this is where I think AA shares such wisdom with The Twelve Steps. The good news here is I think you can learn to navigate life with a little more awareness with just the first five. I've adapted the language of the steps a bit so they apply to everyone, not just people living with addiction.

Step 1. We admitted we were powerless over the vices in our life; that our life had become unmanageable.

We must be ruthless with our inner lives and our vices. Whether it's an addiction to pornography or whiskey, self-loathing or narcissism; whether it's an incessant need for control or a need to be right; whether it's a desperation to be liked or perceived as important—when these vices become unmanageable, the first step to repair is recognizing and admitting we're broken.

Step 2. Came to believe that a Power greater than ourselves could restore us to sanity.

This one requires acknowledging there's something bigger than ourselves. I admit, this one can be challenging. Fortunately, we get to pick what our higher power is. For some people it could be God or an energy. For others it could be a chair or a river. Whatever it is for you, it must be bigger than you. Acknowledging a higher power opens us up to the idea that we aren't the center of the universe.

Step 3. Made a decision to turn our will and our lives over to the care of a higher power as we understood it.

When I was diagnosed with ALS at forty-three, I found a new type of freedom I hadn't experienced before. With a looming expiration date on my life, I felt a bit lighter and less afraid.

I've always had a fascination with birds and their ability to effortlessly glide through the air. In 2019, as we hiked through the snowy Grand Canyon, I spotted the most beautiful raven soaring above. Effortless. Content. Free. No worries and just one mission: to be a raven and glide through the canyon. I was mesmerized by the bird and longed to experience life from its perspective. As I wrote earlier in this book, when I had the opportunity later to go paragliding, I became the raven. Having left all my fears and anxieties behind, I had one job: Surrender. Let go. Be present. Be here now. Free.

Here's where the gold is because turning over our will and our lives in this step is all about surrender.

Step 4. Made a searching and fearless moral inventory of ourselves.

Brutal soul-searching is the name of the game. What are your strengths? What are your weaknesses? What are your secrets, including the secrets you keep from yourself? When are you at your best? When are you at your worst, and why? Dig. Search. Seek. Go for this. It's going to be one of the most difficult things you will do in your life. Don't quit. The best version of you has yet to be seen.

Step 5. Admitted to a higher power, to ourselves, and to another human being the exact nature of our wrong.

Put it out there. Call it like it is. When I was in my early thirties and my friend Herb was around fifty-two, Herb got cancer. Doctors gave him about a year. That year, I went over to Herb's house once a month; we'd sit in rocking chairs on his back porch together and have a cigar. Cigars with a buddy are the best because it's an investment of time. A cigar gives the conversation time to breathe and mature. We'd spend the first third of the cigar shootin' the shit, then the next third moving into more serious matters of the soul, and by the final third, we'd followed the flow of conversation into sacred space. Herb had been sober for a couple of decades. This man, my friend, had lived a hundred lifetimes and was now staring down death. So, I listened and listened and listened some more.

One day I asked Herb, "What is it about you and others I know in recovery? Why are my relationships with addicts so rich and life-giving?"

Herb took a long draw on his cigar, savoring the smoke in his mouth, and slowly exhaled. "It's because we're done bullshitting," he said.

That's it. No more bullshitting. It's time to grow up. No more bullshitting others, and more importantly, no more bullshitting ourselves.

What we have in just these first five of The Twelve Steps is enough to propel us toward positive life change. (I strongly encourage anyone interested to work through the remaining seven steps, which hold incalculable value no matter your relationship to addiction.) Changing the trajectory of your life has more to do with unlearning than with learning. It has more to do with surrendering than acquiring. This is narrow road kind of stuff, and this is why the narrow road isn't as crowded. It is not a path for the semi-committed. This road is the road to life, but it takes you past a million deaths. It forces you to face life on life's terms. To endure hurt and pain and grief. To face your demons and every other part of yourself. As difficult as it is, for those who choose the narrow road, there's no regret.

In life, like in poker, you're dealt a hand. Sometimes you're dealt pocket aces. Sometimes you're dealt a 3, 8 offsuit. You don't get to fold. How will you play your hand? Will you fake your way through it? Will you pretend those aren't your cards? Will you blame the dealer? Or will you accept your hand and get to work? Life is hard. Show up for the game. Allow yourself to be pushed and challenged. Argue with life. Get mad at life. Love it. Curse it. Kick it. Hug it. Embrace it. Learn from it. You got a spot. Claim it. Allow yourself to mature. To grow. To transform. Give yourself and the world your best version of you. And don't ever forget ...

Life is a beautiful clusterfuck and love is here.
Onward. Forward.*
love.

CHAPTER 16

ALS IV

"And in the face of that disease,
When the muscles start to squeeze the life right out of you,
When most men shudder at the dread,
There's this thing you said,
About being the luckiest man on the face of the earth."
—Don Chaffer; The Luckiest Man on the Face of the Earth

April 14, 2023, marked three years with ALS. In my post-trach life, I needed twenty-four-hour care. We now had three part-time caregivers plus Kristy. Our math showed us the numbers: To employ caregivers sixty hours per week, it was costing us $120K per year out of pocket. And I wasn't working. We were living on social security and disability payments. To help with the expenses, Kristy got together with a few friends and launched a one-day fundraiser called Blove 4-14. We asked for $14 donations, and we asked each person who donated to ask ten friends to also donate $14. Thanks to a core group of friends and supporters, and lots of strangers, we raised $116,000 in one day.

Year four was off to a good start. By this time, I had been trached for six months. I was coming out of the fog. I still hadn't found my personal groove, but our family was settling into a rhythm. At the end of April, MK found us another caregiver, an ICU nurse named Gentry. Gentry was another easy hire, with her bubbly personality and desire to learn. I knew Gentry would fit right in when on her second day we took the eight-block stroll to my coffee house. At the first cross street, Gentry, who was driving my chair, took my head in her hands and moved it across my field of vision, and said, "Brian, look both ways."

The only real problem during this era—or perhaps better stated, *my* problem—was a disconnect between Kristy and me. I already missed our pre-ALS dynamic, and now with the hiring of caregivers, we were spending less time together. Whereas we once spent two hours every day showering, now caregivers did that with me. Whereas we once spent an hour on the bedtime routine together, now caregivers were helping me with this too. It was the greatest catch-22. Having caregivers gave Kristy time to breathe and ultimately allowed us to simply be husband and wife again, but we hadn't developed new ways to spend time together.

I wasn't fully conscious of this disconnect until mid-May. For the first three years of ALS, I greatly enjoyed going down memory lane with lots of different friends from high school and college. We would get together to share stories from the past and compare our memories, exploring the similarities and differences. One afternoon I heard a song that reminded me of a high school crush. I asked Kristy if I could text her to go down memory lane. She said she didn't mind. This old friend and I texted back and forth for a few weeks, and the rabbit hole went really deep, really fast. I found myself wanting to check my messages often. At first we just flirted, but then our conversation got more intense. I was reeling her in with my words, and she was reeling me in with her sensuality. I got nervous about where it was going, but I was enjoying the attention too much to stop.

One night as Kristy and I were lying in bed, Zoe Moon walked in and asked, "Mom, why are you crying?" I hadn't noticed her crying. When Zoe Moon left the room, I asked Kristy what was up. She told me that a week earlier while she was running updates on my phone, a message popped up from that friend. Though it was uncharacteristic of Kristy to snoop, she got curious and opened the thread. It crushed her.

This is when I recognized how disconnected from Kristy I'd become, and how lonely I'd been feeling. Which was no excuse but revealed to me why I'd been acting this way and what I was looking for. Kristy had nothing to explain or to say. I'd counseled lots of couples through this kind of stuff, and I told her (and myself) what I said to all of them: "Brian, you fucked up. Your job now is to give Kristy all the space and time she needs. Don't make excuses or even talk. Pull out your phone right now and tell this woman you can't talk anymore. And just to reiterate, you're an idiot."

This is hard to explain, and it might be even harder for some people to comprehend, but in my heart I didn't think Kristy would be upset about my texting relationship. In hindsight, I see my thinking was distorted, but in the moment it felt like I might be relieving Kristy, like she would have one less task on her plate if I flirted with someone else. Needless to say, I read the situation incorrectly. Instead, it broke her. And for a few days I thought I'd broken us. I was completely lost and didn't know what to do. But if Kristy and I are good at anything, we're good at working through difficult situations. We both knew how to express our feelings, we both knew how to listen, and we both knew how to validate the other's feelings without trying to change or minimize them.

Kristy explained that what broke her wasn't the flirting itself but the way I'd used my words to flirt. Having spent years learning how to use words—through reading, writing, and teaching—I'd become a bit of a wordsmith, a poet. "She doesn't get your words. Those are for me," Kristy said, and it instantaneously broke my heart and woke me up. Not to mention that with the limitations of ALS, my words are the only things I have to give away. I'd been careless with my greatest gift. It took us a week, but we worked hard to get to the root of it and figure out a way forward together. And I was more aware than ever of just how big an asshole I'm capable of being.

One of my favorite scenes from one of my favorite movies, *The Wedding Singer*, is when Julia (Drew Barrymore) shows up at Robbie's (Adam Sandler) house to give him a gift of sheet music so Robbie can write his own music scores. He says something really stupid before she has a chance to give it to him, and Julia throws the gift into the air in response. As the papers drift down all over the lawn, Julia says, "You are such an asshole!" and leaves. Robbie bends down to examine the pages, realizes his folly, and says, "I am an asshole!" That was me.

After that week of talking and listening, Kristy ordered us a new queen-size bed. We began working intentionally to spend one hour a day talking, to go on weekly dates, and to sleep in one bed together so we could touch and hold hands. We were connected again, more than ever and stronger together.

At the ALS clinic the next month, I asked Dr. Edwards, who had diagnosed me three years and two months earlier and given me two to five years to live, how long I could possibly live now that I was trached. I optimistically told him I hoped to live to 2030 to see Zoe Moon graduate high school. "Why not 2040 or 2045?" he asked. I was so excited about his reciprocation of my optimism but tempered it with my response: "I need to check on my life insurance policy because I need to die one day before it expires."

In July of 2023, I journaled,

I give all of July a 10/10. Physically. Emotionally. Socially. Mentally. Spiritually. Relationally. It is all good in my soul.

For the first time since my diagnosis in April 2020, I finally feel like myself again. I am building rhythms back into my life such as wake-up times, meditation times, times to write, and times to spend with others and Kristy and the kids.

I recently told my dad that for the first time since diagnosis I finally am starting to feel like myself again. He asked me, "How can you feel more like yourself when you can't move a damn thing?" I didn't have an answer for him and needed to process it.

As I have been thinking about it, I have come to a few conclusions. I am more than my body. Bodies are nice, but I can live and be me without it. In addition, I am content. Three and a half years ago, I could eat and walk and talk and breathe on my own. Now I can't. That was then. This is now. And I won't live my life looking in the rearview mirror. There is too much life ahead of me. So, I can feel like myself again because what I could do with my body did not make me who I am. Those things were mere extensions and expressions of who I am. I am still me without those particular expressions. So, I am myself, only a reborn version.

And honestly, I like my reborn version better.

Originally, my doctors told me I wouldn't make it to forty-eight. Now I say, "Hold my beer. No, seriously, hold my beer. I can't hold it."

Life is a beautiful clusterfuck and love is here.
love.

Along with once again feeling myself and feeling as though I might actually live came some unexpected visitors. I'd spent the first three years of ALS thinking I might not make it to the next day. For three years I lost a little more function every single day. I took nothing for granted. Living in the present was easy for me. My only concern was to be fully present to what or who was right in front of me.

In one of the greatest plot twists of all time, once I hit the nine-month mark post-trach, I realized I might actually live, and just like that everything came rushing back. Worry. Stress. Anxiety. The weight of day-to-day life. I began worrying about our long-term finances and caregiver situation. I began feeling anxious about the kids' college plans and how we would maintain our house. At this point we had three teenage drivers all with cars. Our insurance rate was climbing, and since they all drove old cars, things were always breaking.

I also noticed myself becoming more particular and less patient. MK found us another caregiver in August, a nursing student named Becca, and a few months later, Kristy found another student named Rachel. This marked the first time I didn't hire someone on the spot and instead engaged them on a trial basis. It was a wise decision, of course, and how all caregivers would be hired from that point on. Still, I noticed myself becoming much less patient with the training process. This had nothing to do with Becca, Rachel, or any of the other trainees; something was going on in me. After more than three years with ALS, I understood exactly how I wanted to be cared for, and I had very high standards, so I extended myself a lot of grace as I tried to be more patient.

What I didn't like, though, was the angst I was experiencing. I hadn't felt this kind of weight in years, and it was keeping me from living in the present, a state I'd maintained and enjoyed since my diagnosis. I found myself getting lost in my mind, worrying about the future, and missing out on what was happening right in front of me. Add to this the stress of shifting relationships. As 2023 came to a close, my caregiver situation drastically changed. MK, Britley, and Gentry all left the team, which was incredibly painful for me. The loss of my original team, save Andy, was a difficult time. It's probably impossible for people who haven't worked with a care team to understand, but taking care of a guy who can't move or talk takes incredible time and effort. They knew my eye signals, they knew what I needed before I typed it, and they cared for me as though I were their only priority. Losing MK, Britley, and Gentry was like losing family.

I texted my friend Steve, who has lived with ALS for twelve years, and asked him how he dealt with the loss of good caregivers. He wrote back, "Oh man, fucking fuck dude, I'm feeling this." That's pretty much what it feels like. I loved these girls, and whatever the reasons for their departure, it was difficult for me. I had to come to grips with more loss and the reality that there would be constant turnover in my care. I am grateful to MK, Britley, and Gentry for their dedication to our family, for how, along with Andy, they got us through the first year of life with the trach. I'm especially grateful to Britley and MK for laying the groundwork for all future caregivers. Our second round of caregivers was incredible too, and even provided us with a more holistic approach to what a caregiver could be.

So, why were these feelings and emotions—unexpected visitors—back, and what was I to do with them? After discussing this topic with a friend, he shared the following quote from the French writer René Daumal:

> *You cannot stay on the summit forever; you have to come down again. So why bother in the first place? Just this: What is above knows what is below, but what is below does not know what is above. One climbs, one sees. One descends, one sees no longer, but one has seen. There is an art of conducting oneself in the lower regions by the memory of what one saw higher up. When one can no longer see, one can at least still know.*

I've been to the summit. It was my address for three years. Now I know what it looks like. My desire is to spend much more time there in the future, and I trust I will, but as Daumal says, one cannot stay on the summit forever.

As I reflected, I asked myself two questions and came to many conclusions.

Why are these unexpected and unwanted feelings and emotions back?

Because, life. For three-plus years, I was hanging on for dear life. Doctors said I wouldn't make it to forty-eight, and at times it felt like they would be right, and yet here I am sitting comfortably well into forty-seven. With my trach, I'm stable. Things could still go wrong. I could easily get pneumonia or a blood clot. Perhaps my vent will malfunction or one of my kids will unplug my ventilator to charge their phone or I'll die in a car crash or get cancer. But I'm stable and back in the game of life, and with that comes the daily grind. They snuck up out of nowhere. One day I woke up and there were worry, stress, anxiety, and distraction, and they'd all brought their suitcases. Hello, you pesky old friends.

What am I supposed to do about it?

Everything I've written in this book, naturally. Everything I've learned and practiced over the past three years.

People often ask others as a form of motivation, "If you knew you were going to die at the end of the week, how would you live? What would you do?" I know from experience that it's easy to live when you think you're dying. You don't take one breath for granted, you enjoy every sip of coffee as though it might be your last, you don't want any hug to end, you make sure the people you love know you love them. It's easy to make the last word "love." You take life on its terms, and you relinquish control in order to experience life in your final days.

Yes, it's easy when you think you might die tomorrow. The more difficult question to answer is, "Say you know for certain you'll live tomorrow and for years to come. How will you live? What will you do? Who will you be?"

During my time on the summit, I stumbled upon a teaching by Tilopa, who was a practicing Buddhist in India in the second century. His greatest contribution is what's known as the Six Words of Advice. The six are: Don't recall, don't imagine, don't think, don't examine, don't control, and rest. I know, I know, it's eleven words. Blame the translation.

Tilopa's six words are intended to lead a person to live in the present. "Don't recall" means you shouldn't spend any time thinking about what was. "Don't imagine"—don't bother thinking about what might be. "Don't think"—let go of everything happening right now. "Don't examine"—don't try to figure anything out. "Don't control"—don't try to make anything happen. "Rest"—relax and be present. All of this came easily to me when I was on the summit, but I'm back to practicing. In addition to paying attention to my elbows, I now refer to Tilopa's advice.

Doing life with all of its emotions and stressors is different this time because I've experienced a different, more fulfilling way to live in the middle of the clusterfuck. I've been to the summit, and I know what's possible. I can't say it's easier this time; in some ways it's more challenging because I find myself striving for this summit experience, and striving itself is contrary to the new life. On the summit, there was no striving. Such is life. This is why we train: because life is going to keep coming, and there's nothing we can do to stop it.

ALS might be the greatest thing that ever happened to me besides Kristy and my kids. Its gifts far outweigh what the disease has stolen from me. As of this writing, it has a few things left to take, like the few neck and facial muscles I still have, as well as some internal workings, for example with my lungs and bowels. But for the most part ALS has done what it can to me, and to ALS I say, "I'm still standing, motherfucker!" Well, I'm standing on the inside. And though I think it's done taking, I don't think it's done giving.

What has ALS given me so far?

Perspective

There's nothing like facing your own mortality if you're looking for inner transformation. ALS has reminded me what's really important and afforded me the opportunity to focus on those things. I know who I am and what I'm for. I'm part of the Oneness of love and beauty. I'm a sojourner. My life is for others. I care immensely for the holistic well-being of others, starting with my Kristy and my children, and extending to everyone in my life. I have no agenda other than to give myself to others and walk beside them as they find and begin to live from their soul.

Relationships

Most people don't know how loved they are until their funeral, and then they aren't there to appreciate it. I've experienced how loved I am, I've developed new relationships with many people because of ALS, and I've deepened relationships that were already dear to me. I've also rekindled many relationships of old, reconnecting with old friends. Relationships I wrecked in the past have been completely restored.

Kristy

Kristy and I have gone through a lot in our twenty years of marriage. We had five kids in seven years, including adopting our daughter from Ethiopia. We lost everything we owned in Hurricane Katrina, including our home. We left everything we knew to move to a new city to start a new church with a few friends. All these happenings carried with them extreme highs and lows. In some ways they prepared us for ALS, but then again nothing can really prepare you for the words, "You have ALS." Through ALS, we've experienced a love that I thought only existed in fairy tales. This kind of love is otherworldly.

Kids

My connection with my kids is simply surreal. I was a good kid as a teenager, but I gave my parents a run for their money. When I first got sick, I told the kids, "I don't know how long I have with you, but while I'm here, I'll give the best parts of myself to you. It's up to you whether and how you receive it." All five of our kids handled my diagnosis differently, according to their personalities. As we walked through it with each of them, they grew as individuals even while our family navigated ALS together. Where parent-child friendships usually form as kids leave home, we developed friendships while our kids were still in their teens. At the precise moment they were supposed to be rebelling and pushing limits, they instead responded to correction and discipline with respect. I never imagined a dad and a mom could have true friendships with their teenagers, but here we are.

Time

I was given two to five years to live. This disease forced me immediately into retirement. This afforded me time to devote to the most important things, which included family, neighbors, friends, soul, mind, and living slowly and intentionally.

Curiosity

I've learned to be curious, not judgmental. The truth is, I spent much of my life certain about many things and judgmental of anyone who didn't believe what I believed. I've learned there's nothing scarier than a person who's certain of their beliefs, including religious and political beliefs. Certainty is the killer of curiosity and absolutely the killer of love.

Conversation

Conversation is invaluable, and arguing is futile. Civilized conversation, even regarding disagreements, is an opportunity for restoring relationships—or ending them if necessary, but in a respectful way.

People

Some people are asshats, but for the most part, people are beautiful, incredible, kind, generous, and gracious. People are also hurting and wounded and in need of love. Just like I am.

Life

There's no escaping life. Life is coming for us all. What is this world we live in? There's no rhyme or reason. It just is. We would all do better to cut each other some slack because we're all going through something. Some of us, like me, wear it on the outside. However, many more wear it on the inside where it can't be seen. Years ago now, when I walked out of my doctor's office, I fell to the ground in the corridor. Kristy fell with me, and we hugged and cried together for half an hour. No words. Just tears and embrace. I thought my life was over. Little did I realize my life had just begun.

Magic

The world is full of funk and chaos, and yet at the same time, the world is full of magic and wonder and awe. I've seen newborns who should die make miraculous recoveries. I've witnessed the unimaginable generosity of people. I've seen love in places where I thought love was dead. I've stood in the most powerful thunderstorms, and I've sat beneath magnificent oaks while watching squirrels play and listening to birds sing their praises. The world is a glorious place filled with love and joy and goodness. The world is full of magic.

Love

My heart is full. I'm no saint, so I still don't like or have respect for everyone, but I harbor no animosity or hard feelings. I've adopted a lifestyle of love, and I'm more convinced than ever that regardless of religious beliefs, it's all garbage without love. Religion means nothing without love and acceptance and inclusiveness; without these, it's just a big pile of stinky cow manure. Love is the greatest force in this world. There's nothing love can't handle. There's no problem love can't fix. There's no bond stronger than love. We live in a world where hate and violence seem to be the preferred methods of settling the score. I can think of no greater example of missing the point. When it's all said and done, love wins.

Wisdom

By wisdom, I mean for the first time in my life, I know that I don't know anything—or, as I like to say, I don't know shit about fuck. Life experience is all I have to give. I finally have the wisdom to know that what works for me might not work for you. You must find your own path.

Beautiful Clusterfuck

Life is absolutely beautiful. And life is an absolute clusterfuck. You can't have one without the other. Those who have eyes to see will also find love in the middle of it all. Life is a beautiful clusterfuck and love is here.

As I wrote this chapter, I revisited a scenario that arose in "ALS III": What if a healing man were to walk up to me and ask, "Do you want to be healed?" Back in year three, my answer was, "No, ALS has given me more than it has taken away." Today, I think I'd say, "Show me what you've got." See how I changed and evolved over just a few months? I feel ready to return to work and as a healthy man try my new ways of living. But since I don't think the healing man is coming anytime soon, I intend to remain content and keep learning and growing and loving.

On July 4, 1939, with less than two years left to live, New York Yankees legend Lou Gehrig stood at home plate at Yankee stadium and in front of thousands of fans, teammates, coaches, and opponents delivered a speech in which he said, "For the past two weeks you have been reading about a bad break. Yet today I consider myself the luckiest man on the face of the earth." I resonate with Lou's words and feel them deep in my bones. I wouldn't have chosen ALS, but sometimes you don't get to choose, and ALS has given me life in ways I know I wouldn't have experienced without it.

I stand with Lou as I too consider myself to be the luckiest man on the face of the earth.

My desire, whether I'm here for fifteen more days or fifteen more years, is to continue this journey of the soul and to grow in the ways of love. When I was diagnosed in 2020, I made a conscious decision to devote the rest of my life to the ways of love and continue growing in love. I've spent every single day since diagnosis pondering and practicing love. So, one more chapter.

Life is a beautiful clusterfuck and love is here.
Onward. Forward.*
love.

CHAPTER 17

ON LOVE

> *"The best beggars are choosers,*
> *The best winners are losers,*
> *The best lovers ain't never been loved,*
> *And first place ain't easy,*
> *The hardest part is believing,*
> *The very last word is love."*
> —The Avett Brothers; High Steppin'

One of my favorite stories from the Christian scriptures is about a time Jesus lived in accordance with his teachings on love, forgiveness, and enemy love. Jesus was a man known for speaking truth to power, and one day he was arrested, tortured, and crucified by the powers he spoke up against. Before he died while hanging on a cross, bleeding and gasping for air in excruciating pain, Jesus forgave his murderers. Then, three days later, he rose from the dead. Immediately upon coming back to life, Jesus found the backstabbing friends who'd abandoned him during his persecution, and in otherworldly fashion, Jesus forgave them. He basically said, "Did you get it out of your system? Are we good now? Okay. Cool. I forgive you. Now go in peace, be peace wherever you go, and let's try a new way. The way of love."

For me, this is one of the greatest stories ever told, as it challenges our expectations. Who comes back from being tortured and mutilated and executed and forgives his perpetrators? Who eats with friends who abandoned him in his darkest hour? This is a story of epic love.

What could I possibly add to the volumes that have been written on the subject of love? What do I have to contribute to the poets and artists and music-makers? All I have is my experience, which is of a man who at a certain point decided to devote his life to the way of love.

I like how Alanis Morissette speaks of love in her song, "Sandbox Love." Love, she sings, is

> *Awkward as fuck, precious as fuck,*
> *Sexy as fuck, scary as fuck,*
> *Sacred as fuck, healing as fuck,*
> *Playful as fuck, present as fuck,*
> *Sweet as fuck, here as fuck.*

I also really like Saint Paul's take on love:

> *Love is patient, love is kind*
> *It does not envy, it does not boast, it is not proud.*
> *It does not dishonor others, it is not self-seeking, it is not easily angered.*
> *Love keeps no record of wrongs.*
> *Love does not delight in evil but rejoices with the truth.*
> *It always protects, always trusts, always hopes, always perseveres.*
> *Love never fails.*
> *And now these three remain: faith, hope, and love.*
> *But the greatest of these is love.*

I think both artists were acutely in the flow of Oneness as they wrote. So far none of the couples whose weddings I've had the honor of officiating have asked me to work in Alanis's thoughts—they preferred St. Paul's—but I'm still hopeful.

ON LOVE

As I near the end of my life, I have some wisdom to share on love. For love is the flag I've chosen to plant in the soil of my life. I've chosen to align my motives and my life with love. I've put all my eggs in love's basket. I trust in the deepest part of my being that, when it's all said and done, love wins. And if it doesn't win, well at least it will win in my life, for I've given myself over to a belief that the very last word is love.

The precise moment I chose love is tough to pinpoint, but I began to make steady progress toward love in 2015 when I emerged from a great depression, and I fully committed when I was diagnosed with ALS and received a prognosis of two to five years left to live. Since then, I've come to realize—no, believe—that the only thing worthy of my allegiance, worthy of my devotion, worthy of my life, and the only thing worth dying for, is love. I won't pledge my allegiance to a nation, to an ideology, to a religion, to a book, to a person, or to a flag. Only to love.

It wasn't always this way. On September 12, 2001, I stood in line for more than an hour at my local hardware store to purchase an American flag. When I got home to my third-story apartment, I affixed the flag to my balcony with pride. I was, above all, an American!

Years later, when I had the opportunity to begin traveling the world, my eyes began to open to American imperialism and how others in this great, beautiful world experienced the United States, and it wasn't good. Moreover, as my world got bigger and I interacted with people of other cultures, I realized no people were my enemies—not even the ones I'd been taught were my enemies. It began to look like I'd been taught that anyone different from "us" was a danger and a threat to "us." And if I hadn't been blatantly taught this, the idea was so interwoven into the culture I'd grown up in that I'd definitely absorbed it.

But this us/them way of thinking became too small for me. As residents on the planet, we're all just trying to make it through this life.

We all have good days and bad days. We, as humans, all experience pain and hurt and sadness. We all want to love and to be loved. We all want our loved ones to be safe and cared for. We really are all the same. That became increasingly evident the more I traveled. I searched my soul: Why was I so committed to the country of my birth when there were so many other amazing countries and people on this blue and green ball? I began to feel I'd been duped, indoctrinated, my entire life.

From the age of four, when I entered preschool, I was required every morning to stand, place my hand on my heart, and pledge my allegiance, my life, to this flag, this cause, this one group of people. Whenever we watched the news in our house, we would hear of wars and rumors of war, and how the US was a gift to the world, maybe even a savior. And so, without even thinking about it, at the age of twenty-four, I stood in line for an hour to buy fabric to fly high above my apartment building, ensuring everyone knew where my allegiance lay. I even considered signing up to go kill a bunch of people I'd never met. All because "they" had messed with "us."

9/11 was awful and was orchestrated and pulled off by the most misguided of the human species. At the root of it was *their* indoctrination. But that was no reason for me to build up hate in my heart for entire countries and groups of people. And certainly no reason to sign up to kill. Not for me. So, over the course of a few years and a lot of soul-searching, I changed my mind. Some trust in chariots or tanks; as for me, I'm placing my hope in love.

And just in case my words are taken out of context, I feel the need to add this caveat: I mean no disrespect to the soldiers. But here's the thing. I won the cosmic lottery when it comes to my native country. I was born into the world's greatest superpower. It's as if I were born into 350 BCE Greece when that country was primed to Hellenize the whole world—Alexander the Great, "I will die for you, I will make sure you're safe and we stay at the top of the food chain" Greece. It's as if I were born into 65 CE Caesar-is-Lord Rome, or into the Ottoman Empire in 1638 CE. But I just happened to have been born into today's empire in 1976 CE, and I had nothing, absolutely nothing, to do with it. So, I'm not asking anyone to die for me. I know it will get bad if China or Russia or North Korea becomes a superpower. My skin is crawling just thinking about it, in a way that makes people say, "Sign me up. I will kill for you, my fellow countrypeople. Mr. President (or Madam President), send me."

But the alternative to love has been tried and found wanting; it's not a sustainable way forward. Evil begets evil. Violence desires violence in return. And the cycle continues. We are literally killing ourselves. We are our own destroyers. We succumb to the lie that we can eradicate the darkness with more darkness, even though thousands of generations have gone before us, showing us that it can't be done. The only thing that can dispel the darkness is light. Light one small candle in your pitch-black home as the hurricane outside destroys everything in its path, and within seconds you're able to see the entire interior of your home. One little flame dispels the darkness and the fear. When will we lay down our lives for love? Until we do, I'm afraid we've gone as far as we can go.

I know it feels personal when someone like me speaks out against wars, especially if you haven't considered this way of looking at the issue before, but I suggest that's because we've been taught to identify as a citizen of a country above identifying first as a citizen of the planet. The order is backward. If we recognized our common thread of humanity, followed by our country of origin, I think we would stop feeling the need to kill each other.

Again, I truly don't mean any disrespect toward people who have served, or who are currently serving, in the military. My grandfather served in World War II and the Korean War. I just don't believe any country has the soldier's best interest in mind.

Those paragraphs feel heavy, and I'm not sure I can find a way around it. I think this is where the rubber hits the road. Love is the only thing that can save us. We must wake from our sleep. We must be reborn to see the world as it could be, as it ought to be. The only way to experience this kind of rebirth is through changing our minds and following the way of love. Selling out to the way of love. There's nothing easy about this. It means learning to live with nothing to gain, nothing to lose, and nothing to prove. You no longer have to have the last word or to win every fight. You're free to open your soul to others and their thoughts and ideas. Choosing love is hard, and that's why we don't see more of it. You and I have no control over what others choose. Zero. Nada. None. We can only choose for the one we do have control over.

Choosing love is not a path for people looking for the easy route. The way of love is the way of surrender. To love is to forgive. To love is to admit fault. To love is to choose the other. To love is to lay down your rights for the sake of others. To love is to sacrifice. To love is to choose the well-being of others. To love is to forfeit the need to have the last word. To love is to say, "I am sorry." To love is to set boundaries. To love is to give your vote to someone less privileged than you (this may mean voting against your own self-interest). To love is to say, "I forgive you." To love is to break the rules when love calls for it.

Love is not so much an action as it is an intention. You can do plenty of wonderful things for people and the world, but if you do it without love, it's meaningless on a soul level. You can donate millions, but if your actions lack love, why bother? You can be spiritual AF, but if you're not growing in love, then you're doing it wrong. Without love, actions are like the ridiculously obnoxious clanging sound of dishes when my teenage boys unload the dishwasher.

Love that's true will take you to the highest, most breathtaking highs. Love that's true will also take you to the most devastatingly soul-crushing lows. We are born to love, and then somewhere along the way, we all get stung by someone, and it hurts. We face a choice: Do we choose love, or do we lay the first brick of our wall? When you choose the way of love, you choose to be vulnerable. And with vulnerability comes the potential for pain. We don't always get to choose which comes when, love or pain; we must simply be here for it.

I know, that's a lot of theoretical talk about love. What, you may ask, does love look like in real life? I have a few of those stories. Perhaps you could pour yourself a drink or another cup of coffee.

I met with a family once about their dad's funeral. There were four, maybe five, siblings all in their fifties or sixties. They told me how their dad suffered from dementia in his later years, and how they took care of him in the evenings. One night, he told his boys he was ready to go home.

"But Dad, we are at your home," they said.

"No! I want to go home!"

"Okay, come on, Dad," they said. "Let's go home."

And they loaded him into the car and took him for a drive. They drove past his elementary school, and he pointed to it and talked about his days there. They drove by his high school and the place where he worked for forty-six years, and he reminisced about those places. Then they drove him back home, led him through the door, and helped him settle into his favorite recliner.

"Boys, thank you for bringing me home," he said.

"You're welcome, Pops."

love.

Love is when your father-in-law, in his early thirties, invites his wife's brother, who's the same age and has Down syndrome, to live with him and his growing family. Love is how he then takes care of his wife's brother in every way, from making sure he has a roof over his head and food to eat, to clipping his toenails and helping him shower— and everything in-between. Love is doing this for close to forty years, as Uncle Pete lives to the amazing age of sixty-seven, one of the oldest people to ever live with Down syndrome.

love.

Love is when your friends, who are in their early forties, begin fostering children in the system. Love is their choosing to adopt eight of those children, some of whom have special needs, knowing they will be parenting at least until their late sixties and quite possibly until their dying days.

love.

Years ago, my friend's daughter was stabbed in the hand by another girl in first grade at the local public school. His wife, also my friend, is what we could politely call a spitfire. She met with the school principal about the incident and asked, "What can I do to help?" From there she began a mentoring program, which eventually had as many as fifty mentors, and it's still running twenty-one years later.

love.

Love is when you get sick with a terminal disease and people rally around your family and cook meals. Love is when a friend offers to pay your mortgage for a few years, or when your buddy says he'll get a few people to maintain your house so your wife doesn't have to worry about it.

love.

Stories of love abound. They have the power to transform us if we allow them to.

The sweetest spot is when we ourselves experience love without condition, for this kind of love leaves its imprint on our souls and impacts the trajectory of our lives. Remember: Our lives and souls are only truly transformed through great love or great suffering. And even experiencing great love is sometimes like being forged in the fire.

For me, this kind of transformation through love came around the age of forty-one. I had a childhood friend who remained a dear friend until our early thirties. His wife and I were also close. We got married within a few years of each other and began having children around the same time. One day, I walked away from the friendship.

ON LOVE

No explanation, I just quit. I had my reasons, but I didn't share them. I simply exited their lives and dismissed them from mine.

In my head, my reasons made sense, but in my soul, I knew I was wrong. The truth is, there were things about my friend's wife I didn't like. What kinds of things would drive a person to summarily dismiss not one but two ride-or-die friends? It would have to be something awful, right? Did she stab me in the back? Did she lie to or steal from or slander or cheat me? No. Sadly, it was nothing like that. It even took me years, maybe a decade, to figure out exactly what she did wrong, and figure it out I did: The parts of her I despised were the very things I didn't like about myself. Those traits I hated about myself, well, she possessed some of those same characteristics. In many ways, she was a mirror to my soul. And I drove that train right off the tracks, wrecking decades of friendship, because I was insecure and immature, and I lacked self-awareness. I wrestled with my soul for years until I finally came to a place of humility and was able to name the offense. I called her and asked if she would meet me for a cup of coffee.

As we sat with our coffee, I unpacked for her exactly why I'd mistreated her for the better part of a decade. I apologized and asked for her forgiveness. As I suspected she would, she forgave me. That's the kind of person she is. Then she hugged me and treated me as though I'd never wronged her. Just like that. All was forgiven and gone. I've come to believe that if you care about someone and you got a little love in your heart, there ain't nothing you can't get through together.*

Not long after this experience of unconditional love and forgiveness, I came across a painting in which two individuals embrace in a full-frontal, two-arm hug. One individual holds a bow, and the other has three arrows in their back. For the first time ever, this painting awakened me to the reality that, though I'd taken countless arrows in the back from others, I wasn't blameless. I was myself capable of holding the bow and inflicting unfathomable pain on another. This realization sobered me.

Experiencing the full love from my friend, compounded by the revelation about my own ability to inflict hurt, changed me at a soul level. I was determined to become a master at extending grace. My ability and desire to forgive became a driving force in my life. Humility? You better believe it. I'm capable of hurting others, and now I knew it. Love has the power to change hearts and planets.

Love is when you wreck a dear friendship, and when you get sick years later, the friend you hurt offers to come twice a week to clean your house from top to bottom. Why? Because. Love.

The love I've been writing about here isn't romantic love. I believe in romantic love, as I think I've demonstrated in the pages of this book, but romance muddies the waters. Romance is fickle. For the purposes of this chapter, I'm referring to a purer, platonic love. A love that passes between humans without expectations or strings attached. This kind of pure, platonic love can also exist in romantic relationships.

When I was diagnosed with ALS, I immediately knew what that meant. A life of soon being unable to do anything for myself. I would become one hundred percent dependent on others. Early on, Kristy and I had a conversation about what we were up against. I was devastated that my disease would alter her life in such a significant way. She was only thirty-six years old. I was diagnosed in April, and in July, she surprised me with a vow renewal ceremony during which she re-pledged her love for me, promising she wasn't going anywhere, that she was in it till death do us part.

From there, my health declined quickly. It wasn't long before she had to pick me up and place me in my chair and on the toilet. Within a year and a half, she was bathing me and wiping my butt. By the two-year point, I could no longer move, eat, or swallow; I was completely dependent on others for every aspect of living. Without people, without Kristy, I would have died.

At this time, our kids ranged in age from nine to sixteen. Now, add a 165-pound infant to the mix. Morning after morning, day after day, Kristy got up and did it again. Took care of our entire family. She assumed all the responsibilities that were once mine. She learned how to manage every aspect of our finances, to deal with health insurance and auto insurance and home insurance and mortgage companies and car mechanics and flat tires and house maintenance and getting the dogs groomed—and the list just keeps going. She became an OT, PT, urologist, wheelchair mechanic, changer of feeding tubes, podiatrist, and more. And she was still a mom and a wife, with all the attendant expectations. There were no days off. And she chose to stay. Because that's what real love does. Love lays down its life for the sake of another. Love is a choice. Love is hard. Love costs you everything.

I'm convinced that when all is said and done, no matter what religion, no matter what philosophy, no matter how you choose to live your life, love will have the last word. Whether you worship Allah, God, Yahweh, or the Ocean; whether you follow the path of Jesus, Muhammed, or your great-grandmother Ethel; whether you choose the way of Hinduism or Taoism; whether you're agnostic or atheist—if you aren't growing in love, then you're doing it wrong. You're literally missing the point of life, and you need to change your mind about some things and switch paths. On the other hand, if your heart and soul are growing in love, then whichever path you're on, keep going because you're heading in the right direction.

But I already love my partner and my kids and my friends, so what does growing in love actually look like? I suggest growing in love looks like dropping all of our prejudices, forgiving the wrongs of others, accepting those who are different from us and those we don't understand. Growing in love looks like accepting responsibility, standing with the marginalized, and loving even when it's hard. Loving especially when it's hard.

Love like this is bliss. During my time on the summit, there was nothing anyone could do to sway me from love, though some tried. I didn't seem to meet everyone's expectations of how to approach this disease, and they let me know it. I rarely cursed publicly before ALS (I always loved those words, but I respected my role as pastor). After watching my early video updates, some people gave me a hard time about my use of "motherfucker" and "fuck." I didn't mention faith very often in my updates, so others felt the need to check in with me about my "relationship" with God. Some got sideways with me because I didn't handle situations in my personal life the way they thought I should. As time passed, a few people wrote me off for various reasons, and some people have left in unkind ways. I've had the option to hold on to hard feelings, or to let them go. On the summit, it was easy to love through it all. Forgiveness was automatic. Calm was the natural state of being. Peace and acceptance and grace and mercy and kindness and love were the water I swam in and the air I breathed. On the summit, everything was alive with love—every bird, every tree, every conversation, every conflict. Every thing.

While I'm no longer on the summit, I'm sticking with love. On the summit, I was given an imagination for how life could be best experienced, and now I use that imagination. For this reason, I won't waste days holding grudges or withholding love or being angry. I don't have time for that. I don't know whether I'll wake up tomorrow. So, I'm betting everything on love.

Ultimately, love wins.

Keep chasing love. Pursue it at every turn. Resist the easy way out. Take the high road. Let not hate or anger or judgmentalism or envy or pride or vengeance or arrogance or fear or unforgiveness have the last word. Let love. For love is the only way to live fully. Love is the only way to walk without heavy shoulders. Love is the only way to know a life that is truly free.

When I was a practicing Christian, I daily prayed the prayer of Saint Patrick. I've since adapted the prayer and still pray it every day.

Love be with me; Love within me,
Love behind me; Love before me,
Love beside me; Love to win me,
Love to comfort and restore me.
Love beneath me; Love above me,
Love in quiet; Love in danger,
Love in hearts of all that love me,
Love in mouth of friend and stranger.

For those who have eyes to see, once you commit to love you will begin to notice it everywhere. You will notice love in the embrace of a lover, in the laughter of a friend, in the whistling wind through the great oaks, in the cooing of a baby, in the flutter of a hummingbird's wings, in the tears of a mourning friend, in the face of your pet, in the stars and moon as you gaze upon them. You will find love in the singing of a mockingbird, in the eyes of the barista, in conversation with a friend, in the song on your turntable.

You will recognize love when walking your dog through your neighborhood, in the hug of a stranger, in the birth of a baby, in the flutter of a butterfly, in the joy of a wedding, in the moment of a spiritual service, in the voices of angels, in the grass between your toes, in the quiet of your soul. You will recognize love in every conversation. In every encounter with another. In every encounter with self. Every meal. Every act of lovemaking. Every conflict. Every resolution. Every illness. Every victory. Every defeat. Every encounter with creation. Every life. Every death. Every tear. Every laugh. Every thing.

The universe is alive with love, for love is what binds everything together. Nothing is wasted, everything is sacred, and all of it matters. And somehow, some way, everything will be redeemed in beauty and love, as Oneness weaves the thread of love through every moment, from billions of years ago until now.

Or maybe I'll come back as a bumblebee.

If love is where this whole thing is ideally going, start practicing now. Choose to build your life on love. It will be one of the most challenging endeavors you will ever commit to. It will cost you sweat and tears and relationships and exhilarating highs and excruciating lows. A heart that has not been opened to love cannot be broken, but the heart opened to love, well, that heart is vulnerable to shattering into a billion tiny slivers. This will be difficult, but if you aim to be a person of love, you will build the most beautiful life.

And for all of us, may the very last word always be …

love.

APPENDIX 01

A LETTER TO THOSE I PASTORED

When I was in my early thirties, a dear friend was let go by the church where he'd been an associate pastor for close to twenty years. In his time away from ministry, he took the opportunity to reevaluate his life. This era challenged his faith and led him down paths I didn't understand. His journeying scared me, as I felt my friend and mentor changing his mind on beliefs we'd previously shared.

I think my reaction was normal, though in hindsight I see that I mistakenly thought my friend was losing his faith because something hadn't gone his way. In truth, his faith and life were being stretched. The container he'd been living in for the prior two decades was no longer able to hold his new experiences of love, loss, life, and faith. Something had to give. In Jesus's terms, think of new wineskins for new wine.

As you read the pages of this book, you may assume that my illness caused me to lose my faith. The truth is, however, that my illness prompted me to finally search for and push through answers to questions I'd been asking for years.

I'm not suggesting you follow my lead on this journey. My desire is that you continue your own journey. That said, if along the way my stories stir up questions in your soul, don't run away from those questions; run toward them.

Some of you may get discouraged, concluding I'm no longer a Christian. But if we understand a Christian to be a follower of Jesus (the definition of "Christian"), then that's me: I still adhere to Jesus's teachings on love, forgiveness, nonviolence, anti-nationalism, surrender, enemy love, non-judgmentalism, inclusiveness, serving others, and the many other values Jesus exemplified. I think Jesus was a real historical figure who was committed to a life of love and subversion. I think his teachings are some of the wisest we have access to.

But if we understand "Christian" to mean someone who adheres to Christianity's doctrines, then, no, I'm no longer a Christian. I don't think Jesus is the only way to God; nor do I follow a slew of other Christian beliefs, all of which I unpack in this book.

In the years leading up to my ALS diagnosis, I'd begun gleaning from the teachings of Taoism, Buddhism, Hinduism, atheism, and more. The reason was simple. My life had gotten bigger. My circles had gotten bigger. Some of the people in my life who weren't "Christians" looked more like Jesus than many of the people who identified as Christians. And I reached a point of wondering: Is God so small that in a world billions of years old, God would reveal themselves one time for just thirty years and say, "My way is the only way"? Honestly, God grew too small for me. I don't say that lightly or disrespectfully. I believed the teachings I passed on during my first seventeen years as pastor. Those of you I pastored during the final five years at our church in Midcity—you got the newer version of my thought process.

In the pages of this book, I express my journey. I'm not asking you to follow me if these teachings don't resonate with your soul. I want you to know that when I pastored you, taught you, met with you, and prayed with you, I gave you the best parts of myself as genuinely as possible at the time. But I don't like certainty, and I love questions. I'm inquisitive by nature. Questions don't scare me. Questions fuel me. I'm naturally curious.

I don't regret my twenty-two years of pastoring. I don't regret the person I was. I am the person I am today because of those years, and my hope is that you are more loving because of the time we spent together.

A LETTER TO THOSE I PASTORED

What you hold in your hands could be considered my final sermon.

Thank you for allowing me to speak into your life, some of you for one sermon, some of you for years, and some of you for decades. I hope you questioned everything I taught you, and I hope you were better off in your life because of our time together. Journeying with and pastoring you was one of the greatest honors of my life. Thank you for allowing me that place in your life. My hope for you is the same as it has always been—that your life will be full and light. That you will dance whimsically through life, caught in the flow of beauty, mercy, grace, light, and love.

I love you.

And no matter where life takes you, may the very last word be … love.

—Brian

love.

APPENDIX 02

THE GOSPEL ACCORDING TO TED LASSO*

In 2020, the same year I was diagnosed with ALS, Apple TV released the first of three seasons of *Ted Lasso*. Though it's not a show for every family, it certainly was for us. We piled into the family room on a weekly basis to see what Ted, Beard, Keeley, Rebecca, Roy, Jaime, Sam, Higgins, and the rest of the crew had to teach us. If my kids were ever going to curse correctly, there would be no better teacher than Roy Kent. And it worked. My eleven-year-old daughter knows how to use "fuck" in perfect context with amazing and appropriate inflection.

Ted and his friends showed up week after week to demonstrate true humanity as they navigated the highs and lows of life. They modeled forgiveness and how to say "I'm sorry." They manifested remorse and redemption. They gave us a template for inclusion and acceptance. They exemplified true community and friendship. They taught us how to work through conflict. They showed us how to handle loss and win graciously. Above all, they showed us what love looks like.

The season one finale closes out with AFC Richmond losing its final game of the season in the most heartbreaking fashion and get relegated out of the Premier League. As his players sit stunned and heartsick in the locker room, Coach Lasso delivers his final speech of the season. His words are simple as he talks about how to handle defeat and adversity, and he concludes the speech with an almost throwaway line: "Onward, forward." In the face of demoralizing defeat, he encourages his players to feel it and then move onward, forward. That phrase spoke life to my soul when I needed it most.

To add icing to the Ted Lasso cake, when my eldest son, Micah, graduated from high school in 2023, he immediately took off to Los Angeles to couch surf for a month at the home of a family friend who's a producer. His first week there, he wound up on the *Ted Lasso* set during the shooting of a Christmas special. Micah sat in a hot tub with Brett Goldstein (Roy Kent) and held Hannah Waddingham's (Rebecca Welton) drink while she filmed her parts. One afternoon at the end of shooting, he ran into Juno Temple (Keeley Jones) and told her our family story. Without missing a beat, Juno took Micah to Hannah's dressing room, where they shot a video for me.

During the darkest and scariest three years of our time as a family, Ted and his friends walked through it with us and brought life and laughter and lightness to our weary hearts. *Ted Lasso* is hands down the greatest show I've ever watched twelve times. In our home, *Ted Lasso* is scripture. Every time you see an * in this book, you can thank Ted for that gem.

Onward. Forward.
love.

APPENDIX 03

ALS OUTTAKES

These are stories that don't fit neatly into the book but nevertheless need to be told.

Story #1: I'm Still Standing

Not long after my diagnosis, our family took a road trip. My legs had already stopped working, so I was in my power chair full-time. One of our stops was along the shore of Lake Michigan in Indiana. While the family went for a hike, I parked myself at the top of some stairs overlooking the magnificent lake.

As I sat there enjoying the view and the cool breeze coming off the lake, a man, perhaps in his sixties, made his way from the boardwalk up the stairs. I nodded as he approached and asked, "How are you?" to which he replied, "I'm still standing."

Indeed you are, my good man, indeed you are.

Story #2: War

There are people on every corner asking for money in the part of the city where we live. My practice has long been to roll down my window, shake their hand, ask their name, and give them a few bucks or a sandwich. Most of these people live in a low-income apartment complex for which they use their disability and/or Social Security checks to pay minimal rent. Many are unable to find employment due to their disabilities.

Steve was no exception. As the years passed and I got to know Steve, I often gave him a loaf of bread, turkey, and cheese. Sometimes I pulled over and ate a sandwich with him on the neutral ground. Steve even sometimes came to our church gatherings, always dressed to impress with his slacks, button-up shirt, and tie. We were not that kind of church—I wore pants and a T-shirt—but Steve always showed up spiffy. Steve and I became true friends.

One day Steve called me and said, "Brian, I haven't seen you on the corner in forever. Where are you?"

"Steve, I can't drive anymore. I'm dying. I have ALS," I explained.

The air went silent for a minute. "Well, at least you won't have to see the next big war," he said.

Always the optimist, Steve, always the optimist.

Story #3: Alanis

As I've mentioned, I'm not taken by fame. I am, however, taken by story. What drew me to Alanis was what appeared to be her transformation from the seemingly angsty, hurting, and angry girl that gave the world *Jagged Little Pill* in 1995, into the seemingly peace-filled, healing, and soulful woman that produced *Such Pretty Forks in the Road* in 2020. I love both albums and versions of Alanis. As a society we believe that angst and anger are negative attributes. But are they? Perhaps they are, if channeled in the wrong way, but anger has fueled some of history's greatest movements. Women's rights. Civil rights. LGBTQ rights. Anger has the capacity to destroy the world and to change the world.

The thing about story is that it puts us all on level ground. Once we know one another's story and realize that we all struggle and we all love, we see fewer divisions between black and white, gay and straight, rich and poor, famous and ordinary, American and Iraqi. We just see humanity. Story is sacred.

I don't know what I would be like if I were a zillionaire and an international icon known around the globe by my first name, but I sure hope I would be like Alanis. When we got on our Zoom call in February 2023 (more on that call in "ALS III"), Alanis entered my world for two hours and nine minutes. She didn't once look at her phone during the pauses in conversation as I typed answers to her questions or asked my own. Instead, she engaged in sacred silence with me.

"What did you talk about?" people ask me.

We talked about love, life, soul, spirituality, story, journey, what it means to be human, and more.

"What did she say?" is their next question.

"You'll have to ask her yourself," I say.

About six months after our conversation, I was looking over her tour schedule and saw she would be playing Austin City Limits (ACL). I texted and asked her whether there would be a way for us to connect in person if I made my way to ACL. She texted back that we could connect backstage. So, in October 2023, Kristy, Nate, MK, Andrea, and I headed to Austin.

There was a lot of confusion at the concert. Kristy was on a text thread with Alanis's assistant and tour manager, both of whom were very busy as Alanis prepared to take the stage. We didn't have backstage passes and had no idea whether we were supposed to go backstage before, during, or after the show. The concert started with Alanis dancing across the stage, her voice beautiful and raw, gritty and soulful, spinning in circles, and whipping her head and hair around like she was a six-year-old girl. She's only two years older than I am, and I sure hope I can move like that when I'm her age.

About fifty minutes into an hour-long show, I began to lose hope. As we readied ourselves to leave, we received a text to wait for Alanis's tour manager at the backstage entrance. After half an hour of waiting, I finally told Nate, "When I say go, just drive my chair.

Don't make eye contact, and act like we belong." At that moment the two security guards in the vicinity began chatting with each other. "Go!" I said. We rolled right past them, leaving the girls behind. About fifty feet down the path, we ran into tour buses, more gates, and several more security guards.

Shit.

"What now, Sherlock?" Nate asked.

Moments later, MK and Kristy showed up with the tour manager.

"When will you learn to stop doubting me?" I asked Nate.

The tour manager took us back to the tent for family and friends. Remember that Alanis had just finished performing for thousands of people, and lots of people in the tent vied for her attention. When Alanis eventually found us, she walked right past me and straight to Kristy, giving her the tightest hug. We met her kids and one of her closest friends. We talked for about twenty minutes as her kids ran around and the youngest one tugged on her shirt, "Mommy, Mommy, Mommy."

This was the same woman I had Zoomed with nine months prior. No pretense. No bullshit. No ego. Just kindness and humility and soul and love.

As I neared the end of writing this book, I had some questions for Alanis. I texted her one day and asked if we could FaceTime. "Absolutely," she said. "I'll have my assistant text Kristy to set a time." I prefer to look at it like her assistant texted my assistant, but Kristy doesn't find that as funny as I do.

What I love most about Alanis is her humanity, her groundedness, her ability to be present, her empathy, and her love. She took time to see me and enter my world. A guy who isn't taken by her fame and didn't want to talk about her music but rather about deep life and soul issues, and her life journey. And she was there for it. Unreal. Most people probably think music is Alanis's gift to the world, but I believe Alanis is her gift to the world. The world is full of magic, and people are amazing.

Story #4: Slurring My Eyes

I've always enjoyed the occasional overindulgence of alcohol, particularly bourbon or tequila. Once I could no longer swallow, I thought my drinking days were over. Ah, but I quickly learned we could just put the alcohol in my feeding tube. I did this a few times and thoroughly enjoyed myself, although the first time I got drunk post-trach and was fully reliant on my computer to communicate, well, that changed the game.

We were on a beach trip, and it was time for our family Texas Hold'em game. I asked MK to give me two shots of vodka through my feeding tube. I wasn't feeling anything after a while, so I asked for two more. Forty-five minutes later, I still wasn't feeling anything, so I asked for one more. When I still couldn't feel the effects of the alcohol, it dawned on me: I wasn't moving. I asked MK to unbuckle me and move my body around. Holy shitballs! Within ten minutes, the room was spinning, and I was out of my mind. At first I thought it was great, but then my eyes started slurring. I could no longer play the game because my eyes would type "I waith fitty dowas," or "MK, I nee a bwanket," and no one could understand me.

My drunkenness increased with each passing minute. When it was time for bed, MK rolled me to my room and began the process. My neck was in great pain because of the way I was positioned. I tried to tell MK, but she didn't understand that "iythkh rtopkz htwdsq" meant "my neck hurts."

And that was the last time I ever drank.

Story #5: The Bumblebee

When he was seventeen, Micah and I had a conversation about what an afterlife might be like.

"I may return as a bumblebee," he said.

I thought that was an odd choice and asked him why. He explained he'd taken that line from one of his favorite movies. In his own words:

In the film Mr. Magorium's Wonder Emporium, *when Mr. Magorium is asked where he's going, as he plans to leave the world in a couple of days, he replies, "I may return as a bumblebee." Over the years that line has worked its way into my speech. The sheer optimism Mr. Magorium has for his next phase truly reminds me of my dad. Like Mr. Magorium, Dad has a unique outlook on life, finds joy in the places many people overlook, inspires others, and embraces the full spectrum of his journey with abiding love. He's able to find beauty, love, humor, and connection within the struggle and pain.*

The bumblebee, a symbol of whimsical acceptance, hope, community, and love, embodies how Dad lives his life and impacts others.

The bumblebee invites and inspires us all to join with my dad, living life with intention, presence, and love.

Micah drew a special version of a bumblebee, and on his eighteenth birthday, Micah, Kristy, and I tattooed the bumblebee on our bodies. When each kid turns eighteen, if they want it, they can get it too.

Story #6: 55 vs 16

1990, freshman year of high school. Mrs. Taliancich was a quirky teacher, but at ninety words a minute she could type like no one I'd ever seen. And she taught me how to type—on a typewriter. I haven't once used the Pythagorean theorem or the periodic table of the elements since high school, but I've used my typing skills every single day. So you see, high school was worth it. I could type fifty-five to sixty words per minute by the time I completed that class, a skill I maintained until the age of forty-four. Once I could no longer use my hands and was limited to writing with my eyes, that number dropped to sixteen words per minute. And that's the speed at which I wrote this book.

Story #7: Chasing Butterflies

Kristy's bestie is Andrea. Andrea is easy to love, so she and I have also been friends for more than fifteen years. To understand these stories, you need to know a little bit about Andrea. For starters, she brings the fun. She brings the glitter and the pizzazz, and in her next life she'll probably return as a unicorn. Andrea is the kind of person who doesn't meet a stranger, and she's also a bit ADD and easily distracted. So, if you're walking with her and she sees a butterfly, whatever you were talking about vanishes, and you probably just lost your walking partner too because now she's chasing butterflies.

One evening we had a few friends over, and I asked Andrea to assist me to the back porch and to light my joint for me so I could smoke. At this time, my legs and arms didn't work. It was a cold night, probably about forty degrees. We were hanging out and having a good time when she said she needed to go to the bathroom. "Do not forget me. Go straight to the bathroom and come right back," I told her. About thirty minutes later she returned, and as she opened the door to the porch, I heard, "Oh shit, I got caught up talking and totally forgot about you."

A few months later, Kristy, Andrea, and I took a trip to Austin to see Kristy's other bestie, Liz. One day Kristy went out with Liz while Andrea and I hung out together. We decided to stroll the streets and find some lunch, so Andrea wheeled me to the hotel elevator, got us situated in the elevator, and pressed the down button. When the elevator arrived at the lobby, Andrea got off. I don't know, maybe she thought it was a magic elevator and that I'd magically gotten better on the ride down. Who knows what was going through that unicorn brain, but as the doors closed with her on the outside and me inside, I could see on her face that she realized her folly. Because I couldn't move my arms to press the buttons, the elevator took me to the top floor and then slowly made its way back down, picking up new passengers on each floor.

Butterfly!

Story #8: Nose Goes

Someone recently asked what it's like to be in the Jeansonne family. To understand my explanation you need to understand the game Nose Goes. In Noes Goes, when someone asks for something, each player puts one finger on their own nose. The last person to touch their nose has to do the requested task. Nose Goes isn't something you sit down to play intentionally; it's a spontaneous game. For example: Say you're all settled in and comfortable for family movie night, and five minutes into the movie Mom says, "I want popcorn." Now, the last person to touch their nose has to get Mom's popcorn. Or perhaps we're deep into family game night and I say, "Cough." The last one to touch their nose has to cough me using my cough assist.

If you really want to know how Nose Goes is played in the Jeansonne household, imagine my trach popping off because it wasn't snapped on tightly enough, and then imagine that instead of immediately jumping into action, the family first plays Nose Goes because they know I can hold my breath for ninety seconds.

We're far from a perfect family. We're certainly the most eclectic family I've ever encountered. Our kids don't look much alike, and they don't share the same passions. I sometimes tell Kristy that our four biological sons are as different from each other as they are from their sister who hails from the great country of Ethiopia. I don't know that these five individuals would ever run together, except if they were forced together as they have been. Kristy and I chose each other, and then we chose to make more people, and those people didn't choose to be in the same family. This family was forced upon them. *We* didn't even choose them in particular. Well, we did choose Zoe Moon. I used to tell the boys, "Fellas, the truth is we were stuck with you knuckleheads, but we chose her, so the joke's on you."

The point being, we might not have chosen each other, but we choose each other now.

As I tell the kids, "Now look, this is a sad moment right here, for all of us. There ain't nothing I can say sitting in front of you right now that can take that away, but please do me this favor, will you? Lift your heads up, look around this room. You know, look at everybody else in here. And I want you to be grateful that you're going through this sad moment with all these other folks because I promise you there is something worse out there than being sad. And that is being alone and being sad. Ain't nobody in this room alone. Let's be sad now, let's be sad together, and then we get back up. Onward. Forward."

Yeah. that's what it's like to be part of #thejeansonne7.

Life is a beautiful clusterfuck and love is here.
Onward. Forward.*
love.

ACKNOWLEDGMENTS

I would like to acknowledge my eyes. Writing a book is difficult. Writing a book with your eyes is even more difficult. These eyes just kept showing up day after day, and for that I am grateful.

I would also like to acknowledge...

Windows. I've been an Apple guy for twenty-plus years. Apple, however, does not play well with others and is behind the game when it comes to progress. Windows, on the other hand, is great at playing with others, which is why guys like me can still talk and even write a book.

My rest-of-my-life partner, ALS, for giving me the opportunity to grow and mature and explore more deeply—myself, my life, the big questions. It's been a wild ride, and if at any point you would like to change your mind and leave my body, I'm cool with that.

My suppliers, whom I won't name since we are teetering on illegal activity (but you saints know who you are), who so selflessly shared their Adderall with me after insurance denied my prescription. These are the unsung heroes for how they enabled me to stay awake and focused.

My wife, my friend, my person, my Kristy. For encouraging me to keep writing even when I didn't want to. For reading the same chapters over and over again. For your willingness to drop whatever you were doing to print something for me or reboot my computer when it froze. And for your input. But most of all, for showing me and the world what real love is. You are the most wonderful thing that's ever happened to me. Thank you for your love. love.

My kids. Micah, Jonah, Nathan, Lucas, and Zoe Moon, you are my reasons for continuing this journey. You are my heart. Thank you for giving me the space to write. You guys would walk into the room while I was writing and say something like, "Keep writing, Dad. I just wanted to say hi." Each of you also served as a sounding board for different parts of the book and participated in the writing by giving me your perspective. I can think of no other accomplishments that compare to giving my life for you. Now, fly. love.

Everyone who helped by pulling a book from my shelf and reading passages aloud to me or typing out highlights I needed from other books or typing out my wedding vows and emailing them to me. Anything to make my work a little easier. The people who assisted me in these ways include Andy, Jonah, Micah, Lucas, Nate, Britley, Gentry, MK, and of course, Kristy.

Andy, one of my closest friends, for listening to my playlist ad nauseam while I wrote for hours on end while occasionally needing cough and suction. We now share a great distaste for a good number of songs.

My friend, Steve. For following your professional dream, which was to play a game, as an adult, for a profession, and entertain people like me. Oh, and Steve, thank you for blocking that punt in 2006—I was certainly entertained. For starting Team Gleason when you were diagnosed with ALS. Because of you, I have access to the technology that allowed me to write this book. But most of all, thank you for being my friend.

My friend, Crispin, for reading my original manuscript and giving me feedback, some of which I used. For being a fellow sojourner on this journey of life for close to thirty years. For smoking herb with me once a week for two and a half years, until I couldn't smoke any longer. We hashed out many of the thoughts contained in this book while sitting on Margo's porch. Thank you for being a witness.

Covid. For your impeccable timing. You shut the entire world down so my family and I could spend the first eighteen months of my diagnosis with no sports, nowhere to be. In many ways you were

ACKNOWLEDGMENTS

a jerk, killing people and shuttering small businesses. But if you were inevitable, then you picked a good time for us.

My dear friend, Emily. Thank you for your love and compassion and friendship. Because of you, my transition from speaking for a living to losing my voice and needing a computer to talk for me was smooth, and you made it less scary and actually doable.

My friend, Liane. Originally, every chapter began with lyrics. You worked tirelessly to secure permissions. Thank you for your efforts. Who knew it would be so difficult and so expensive to use lyrics?

A huge thank you to Anders Osborne, Alanis Morissette, Don Chaffer, The Avett Brothers, and The Wood Brothers for graciously granting me permission to use their lyrics for free. While many artists typically charge a minimum of $300 up to $1,000, these soulful and generous artists offered their support without hesitation. Please do me a favor and check out their amazing work!

The most amazing doctor I've ever met, Dr. Kantrow. For your love and support and empathy and friendship. Thank you for your cell number and for always responding. Most of all, thank you for doing everything in your power to keep me around. Stephen, you are an even better man than you are a doctor. Thank you for being you and sharing yourself with the world.

The wonderful Dr. Edwards who gave me two to five years to live, and then encouraged me to live past my life insurance. I would not want your job, Chris, but I'm glad there are people like you who can do it. You are amazing at your job. I can't think of anyone I'd rather have deliver such horrible news and then walk through it with me. I appreciate you.

My summit friend, Micah. You're the only other person I know who has been to the summit and come back down. Our conversations hold a place deep in my soul, and many of them helped me find the language for this book.

My beta readers and my friends, Rachel, Taryn, and Chad. Thank you for the time and energy you invested in this project as you pored over these pages and gave me valued input.

My best friend, my dad. For supporting my journey. Thank you for reading this book numerous times and giving your input, and thank you for always having my back and being my biggest fan. You're the real deal when it comes to integrity, character, open-mindedness, and love. Thank you for giving me the space I needed to make my own journey. You're the best man I've ever known. I hope to be half the man you are when I grow up.

My faithful supporter and chef extraordinaire, my mom. Thank you for always supporting and encouraging and loving me. Thank you for always doing the absolute best you could, and for always loving me and our family of four. Thank you for teaching me the single most important lesson of life when I was sixteen: presence. This book would not be possible without you.

My friend, Faith. Thank you for connecting the impossible dots to get me to Alanis. You pulled a rabbit out of your hat, and your magic trick resulted in a relationship that has enriched my life deeply. Thank you. I owe you one.

My friend, and in many ways a mirror to my own soul, Alanis. Thank you for taking the time to get to know me. Thank you for your encouragement. Thank you for furthering my theory on parallel universes. I'm fairly certain that ALS killed me in another universe, after which I was thrust into this universe where I have an amazing family, am deeply loved, wrote a book with my eyes, and we are friends. Perhaps more than anything, thank you for seeing me.

My editor and now friend, Sara. I think it took you two conversations and three chapters to get me, my sense of humor, my tone, and my message. You made the whole process fun and exciting, and in the end you made this book more than it was when I sent it to you.

My brother, Nathan, you inspire me. You taught me how to ask better questions and how to listen. Our friendship is one of the most cherished things in my life. I raise a glass to you, of anything but TX whiskey. Thank you for being a witness.

My ride or die companion, Luna. My dog. You still don't understand why we don't go on walks or why I don't rub your belly, but that doesn't stop you from loving me. You were with me every step of the way while I wrote this book, spending countless hours on my lap while I worked. I never knew I could love an animal this much. You are getting up in age, so our people in this home are making bets on which of us will outlast the other. I keep telling the kids to put their money on me.

My friend, Jenn, thank you for lending me your photography skills and capturing the images for my cover.

My lifelong friend, Jon, thank you for making my vision for the cover come into existence and most of all for your friendship. I have not always been a good friend, but you have. You have shown me what true love and friendship are. Thank you, Samwise.

My guy, Ted Lasso, and everyone who brought the show named for him into existence when our family needed it most. We laughed. We cried. We learned. And we were inspired.

And last but certainly not least, Vinny, my ventilator. We've been through a lot together. Our relationship is a symbiotic one in that I help you fulfill your purpose on this earth by giving you a set of lungs to fill with air, and you give me the air I need to fulfill my purpose. Without each other, we would both be wasting away, you on a shelf and me in an urn. So, here's to you, Vinny, and to many more years together.

love.

ABOUT THE AUTHOR

Brian Jeansonne is a native New Orleanian and a lifelong student of religion, metaphysics, and philosophy. Brian holds a degree in psychology from the University of New Orleans and received his certification as a spiritual director through Sustainable Faith.

Brian began his career as a pastor, serving for twenty-one years while continually seeking answers to profound questions. In 2020, he decided to step away from pastorship to work more intimately with fellow sojourners as a life coach and soul care director. This life-changing choice coincided with his ALS diagnosis. Today, he spends his working hours writing at a pace of sixteen words per minute, using his eyes, often accompanied by his dog, Luna, in his lap.

Brian lives in New Orleans with the rest of The Jeansonne 7—Kristy plus their five kids: Micah, Jonah, Nate, Lucas, and Zoe Moon.

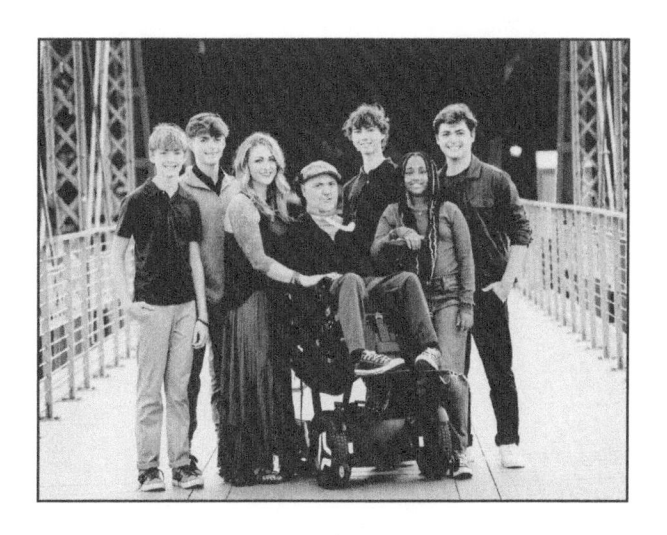

Printed in the United States
115141LV00003B/73/A